FOOL-PROOF WEIGHT-LOSS TIPS

PREVENTION'S BEST™
America's #1 Choice for Healthy Living

FOOL-PROOF WEIGHT-LOSS TIPS

By the Editors of *Prevention* Health Books

RODALE

ST. MARTIN'S
PAPERBACKS

The information in this book is excerpted from *Foolproof Weight Loss* (Rodale, 2000).

Prevention's Best is a trademark and *Prevention* Health Books is a registered trademark of Rodale Inc.

FOOL-PROOF WEIGHT-LOSS TIPS

© 2001 by Rodale Inc.

Cover Designer: Anne Twomey
Book Designer: Keith Biery

ISBN 0–312–97880–4   paperback

Printed in the United States of America

Rodale/St. Martin's Paperbacks edition published November 2001

St. Martin's Paperbacks are published by St. Martin's Press, 175 Fifth Avenue, New York, NY 10010.

10 9 8 7 6 5 4 3 2 1

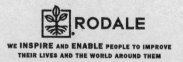

RODALE

WE INSPIRE AND ENABLE PEOPLE TO IMPROVE
THEIR LIVES AND THE WORLD AROUND THEM

JoAnn E. Manson, M.D., Dr.P.H.
Professor of medicine at Harvard Medical School and chief of preventive medicine at Brigham and Women's Hospital in Boston

Terry L. Murphy, Psy.D.
Assistant clinical professor in the department of community health and aging at Temple University and licensed clinical psychologist in Philadelphia

Susan C. Olson, Ph.D.
Clinical psychologist, life transition/psychospiritual therapist, and weight-management consultant in Seattle

Mary Lake Polan, M.D., Ph.D.
Professor and chair of the department of gynecology and obstetrics at Stanford University School of Medicine

Lila Amdurska Wallis, M.D., M.A.C.P.
Clinical professor of medicine at Weill Medical College of Cornell University in New York City, past president of the American Medical Women's Association, founding president of the National Council on Women's Health, director of continuing medical education programs for physicians, and Master and Laureate of the American College of Physicians

Carla Wolper, M.S., R.D.
Nutritionist and clinical coordinator at the Obesity Research Center at St. Luke's–Roosevelt Hospital Center and nutritionist at the Center for Women's Health at Columbia-Presbyterian/Eastside, both in New York City

Contents

The Eternal Quest

Diet. Like other four-letter words, it's one we should banish from our vocabulary. Diets are painful, annoying, difficult, and demeaning—worse, they typically don't work forever. After all, you can't spend your entire life denying yourself your favorite foods for the sake of calories.

So if you're looking for a calorie-counting, rice cake approach to weight loss, you'll have to go elsewhere. If, however, you're looking for a way to revolutionize your lifestyle to incorporate good health and healthy eating—with weight loss as a guaranteed by-product—then you've come to the right place.

In this book, we'll take a deliberately holistic view of weight. It's not about pounds of flesh but how we feel about ourselves and our lives, how we cope with stress and surprises, how we move through our days and nights. Most important, it's about learning to accept ourselves as we are—accentuating our inner and outer beauty, which have nothing to do with any number on a scale.

There is no quick fix to an unhealthy lifestyle, of course, so use this book as if it were a road map for your journey to good health. You can move along as quickly or as slowly as you like, taking what you need from each chapter and discarding the rest. Along your journey you'll find we've jammed this book with the practical and the doable—everything from how to dine in fancy restaurants and still eat right to how to burn extra calories without working up a sweat. We bust every excuse you've ever had about why you can't change, and we tell you how even the people you love the most can sabotage your efforts.

We do all this with help from dozens of experts, including the weight-loss gurus from TOPS—the acronym for the nonprofit group Take Off Pounds Sensibly. It was founded in 1948 by a homemaker named Esther Manz. It's the oldest major weight-control organization in the United States, and with 275,000 members, it's also one of the largest. Its basic philosophy is that to change behavior, you need three things: motivation, skills, and support.

This book provides you with all three.

PART ONE

Getting in Tune
with Yourself

Our Lips Are Sealed— Or Are They?

Any seasoned veteran of the fat wars can recite the basic formula for weight loss as fast as her phone number: Eat fewer calories than you burn. Still, we're always looking for a magic formula to get the job done quickly.

Maybe that's why so many of us dive into diet after diet—on average, about twice a year—before we're prepared to make the permanent lifestyle changes essential to lasting weight-loss success.

"Most people *think* they're ready to lose weight," says Sandra Haber, Ph.D., a New York City psychologist who specializes in women's weight issues. "Yet changing our health habits is a very complex, three-dimensional task, which has been foolishly simplified by standard diet formulas and remedies. The question should be: 'Are you *really* ready to lose weight?'"

Put another way, "Are you *really* ready to change?"

Research shows that permanent health behavior changes occur in five specific stages, says Carol Boushey, Ph.D., assistant professor in the department of foods and nutrition at Purdue University in West Lafayette, Indiana. The so-called stages of change were defined in the early 1990s to help people overcome high-risk behaviors such as smoking and alcohol abuse. Each stage represents a different mindset in the change process.

Experts agree that if you can identify and understand the importance of each stage and learn how to use specific

Are You Ready to Change?

Weight loss involves changing both the number of calories you take in and the number of calories you burn. Too many people commit to one strategy but not the other. Here's how to gauge your readiness to alter your eating habits as well as your activity level. Pick the answers that best describe your mindset right now.

Are you ready to eat right?

A healthy diet means at least five servings of fruits and vegetables, six servings of grains, two servings of lean meat or legumes, and at least two servings of calcium-rich low-fat or nonfat dairy products daily. It also means that you limit high-fat and high-sugar foods.

1. I don't currently eat a healthy diet, and I don't plan to start.
2. I intend to adopt a healthy diet in the next 6 months.
3. I've started making some healthy changes to my diet.
4. I regularly eat a healthy diet, but high-fat, high-sugar foods tempt me now and then.
5. I have been eating a healthy diet for more than 6 months, and it has become second nature to me.

strategies that are effective in each, you'll dramatically boost your chances of progressing from stage to stage and achieving your goals. That's why short-term diets fail, says Dr. Boushey. They ignore your need to progress gradually through these stages.

It will take time. Some people sail through each stage without a hitch. Others might think about starting an ex-

Are you ready to get moving?

"Physically active" means your exertion level equals that of a brisk walk, climbing stairs, or digging in the garden and that you accumulate at least 30 minutes of this level of activity 3 to 5 days a week.

1. I don't exercise, and I don't plan to start.
2. I've been thinking about becoming more active but just can't get started.
3. I exercise once in a while but could do more.
4. I've started exercising regularly, but it's still tough to keep up.
5. I've engaged in regular physical activity for more than 6 months, and it has become second nature to me.

Scoring

Note the number you picked in each area. That tells which stage you're in so you can target your efforts toward your fitness goals.

1. Precontemplation
2. Contemplation
3. Preparation
4. Action
5. Maintenance

ercise program for years before actually lacing up a pair of sneakers. More common is the woman who makes several attempts at change before finally achieving her goals.

In general, if you are willing to make a serious attempt to change, you will probably spend a couple of months at each stage.

The first step is to determine how ready you are to change your eating and activity habits. Once you've identified your readiness level, you can start building new skills that move you toward the permanent lifestyle changes that result in weight loss.

Precontemplation: Why Choose to Lose?

Stage 1: You're not thinking about change at all.

In this stage, you're either unaware of a need for or uninterested in change, says Bess H. Marcus, Ph.D., associate professor of psychiatry and human behavior at the Brown University Center for Behavioral and Preventive Medicine in Providence, Rhode Island, who pioneered the use of stages of change to help people become more physically active. You don't see how losing weight will impact your life. You could be in denial about the health risks of being overweight and inactive. Or you could simply be worn down by repeated dieting failures. People tend to stay at this stage for a long time—sometimes for life—because it feels safe and familiar.

Your wakeup call may come from friends and family's hinting that you need to lose weight, begin exercising, or otherwise change your lifestyle. Your goal at this point is to stop tuning them out and start opening your mind to the idea that change might be good for you.

Knowledge is power. Read, rent informative videos, or surf the Internet to gather health information. Consult your doctor, a registered dietitian, or a personal trainer.

The Big Weight-Loss Myth

It's not true that 95 percent of those who lose unwanted pounds gain it all back—and then some. That figure "doesn't apply to most people," says Suzanne W. Dixon, R.D., a research epidemiologist and registered dietitian at the Henry Ford Health System in Detroit. It springs from a 1959 study of 100 people who were given a diet but no exercise or behavioral modification support. Later, similar studies helped solidify that misleading figure.

"These early studies were conducted among people in clinical programs, using extreme diets, like 800-calorie diets," Dixon relates. "These people were obese, not just overweight, their whole lives. Some had medical issues and problems with compulsive eating. They were not the typical population."

So how many people really do succeed at maintaining weight loss? The National Weight Control Registry (NWCR) is working on an answer. This database of successful weight losers examines a large, general population that has maintained substantial weight loss. Operated by the University of Colorado at Boulder and the University of Pittsburgh, it's collecting information from those who have lost at least 30 pounds and maintained that loss for at least 1 year.

So far, half the people enrolled have lost weight and kept it off. On average, participants have lost more than 60 pounds and maintained a 30-pound weight loss for about 5 years.

Research indicates that those who succeeded had tried to lose weight several times before finally finding what worked, Dixon says. Then they continued to follow low-fat, moderate-calorie eating habits. And they never quit exercising.

This process will open your conscious mind to the idea of change, says Dr. Boushey.

Discover the benefits. Even very modest weight loss—just 5 pounds—can improve how you feel and how your body functions, according to a Harvard study of more than 40,000 women. Conversely, adding too many pounds raises your risk of diabetes and heart disease. To quickly assess your degree of potential health risk, calculate your waist-to-hip ratio. Simply measure your waist (1 inch below your navel) in inches and divide it by your hip measurement in inches. For women, a waist-to-hip ratio of 0.80 or more is associated with increased health risks.

Forget bad experiences. More than 90 percent of those in the National Weight Control Registry—a group of some 800 people who have kept 30 pounds off for at least a year—tried to lose weight several times before they were successful. In fact, on average each had lost and regained a total of 270 pounds. This yo-yoing turns off many people to the thought of starting another weight-loss program. But there is a way around it: Instead of viewing previous weight-loss attempts as failures, consider them a rich source of information of what has and hasn't worked for you, says Dr. Haber. For instance, if eating three servings of fruit a day helped squelch your urge for sweets last time but cutting out dessert entirely induced binges, go back to eating fruit and add a single serving of dessert two or three times a week.

Contemplation: The Wheels Are Turning

Stage 2: You recognize that there's a need to change, but you aren't quite ready to do anything about it.

The focus starts to shift inward, and you begin to evaluate your own behavior and identify habits that you'd be willing to change. Your goal in this stage is to consciously make the decision to change. You'll know you're ready when you're focusing on the solution and the future rather than on the problem and the past.

"There are a lot of changes to contemplate," explains Dr. Haber. "There are changes, for example, in how you set up your home, in what foods you keep in your fridge and pantry, and in the kind of meals you have."

This period of thought and reflection is crucial. Resist the temptation to skip ahead. "You're looking for reasons that will make changing important to you," says Dr. Boushey. "If you jump in too fast, you'll fail because you are not ready yet." Don't move to a higher stage until you've achieved maintenance in the previous stage.

Know your motives. Evaluate your reasons for wanting to lose weight. Are you trying to please your spouse? Slimming down for a class reunion? Trying to lower your blood pressure? Or are you just trying to look and feel better?

"The decision to lose weight is strictly an individual matter," says Kristi Ferguson, Ph.D., associate professor of community and behavioral health at the University of Iowa College of Public Health in Iowa City, who has explored whether our reasons for losing weight influence our chance of success. Researchers analyzed answers from 100 successful and 40 unsuccessful dieters and concluded that it doesn't really matter what your reason is for wanting to lose weight. What matters is where that reason comes from.

"We're more likely to succeed when our motivation comes from within—when we lose weight for ourselves, not to please others," says Dr. Ferguson.

Before you can move beyond just thinking about losing weight to actually committing yourself to a healthy lifestyle program, the positives of weight loss have to outweigh the negatives.

Take Tips from TOPS Club

Its name says it all: Take Off Pounds Sensibly. TOPS Club doesn't offer any quick fixes. Losing weight is up to you. But weekly TOPS chapter meetings can provide the encourage- ment you need to stick with your plan over the long haul.

"I believe that to change behavior, you need motivation, skills, and support," says Howard J. Rankin, Ph.D., behav- ioral psychology advisor to TOPS Club and author of *7 Steps to Wellness*. "TOPS works because it is a support group."

This nonprofit group was founded in 1948 and is the oldest major weight control organization in the United States. With 275,000 members, it's also one of the largest.

Although TOPS endorses a basic dietary exchange pro- gram, it leaves the choice of personal diet and exercise

Think small changes. Making big changes is like trying to swallow a watermelon whole. Instead, pinpoint indi- vidual habits or behaviors that you want to change and why, says Dr. Boushey. For instance, instead of saying, "I'm going to eat less fat," you might decide to switch from whole milk to skim milk. "Set a goal that's realistic and that you can achieve in a short amount of time. Meet it, then pick a new goal," says Dr. Haber.

Recognize your barriers. Think of all the reasons you haven't lost weight in the past: "I don't have time to exer- cise. My family doesn't like diet food. Fresh fruits and veg- etables cost more money." These are barriers—reasons *not* to change. To conquer your barriers, learn the difference between an excuse (I don't have time to exercise) and the real reason (I don't want to get up early to work out). Then find ways to resolve those real reasons, says Dr. Marcus.

program up to you and your physician. TOPS provides lively meetings, motivational materials, and incentives to keep you going.

"People identify with the kinship and friendship that they find at TOPS," says Dr. Rankin. "There is a certain element of feeling just like a club. The fact that everyone there is struggling with the same problems is phenomenally powerful."

If you decide to try TOPS, finding a meeting close to home should be easy. There are more than 11,000 held each week. Your first meeting is free. If you join, annual membership is just $20 in the United States and $25 in Canada. To learn more about TOPS, call (800) 932-8677 or check www.tops.org.

Preparation: Map Your Route

Stage 3: You're ready, willing, and planning to change.

Once you move into preparation, change is no longer a far-off goal. "You can aggressively start to take action," says Dr. Boushey.

Say you're planning to dive in headfirst within the month. To test the waters, you'll probably start exercising once or twice a week and begin making small changes in your eating habits. You may even have a personal trainer, nutritionist, or program specialist to help you.

Once you have a detailed, solid plan of attack, you're good to go.

Plan a reasonable strategy. The key to successful weight control is choosing a plan that is doable, says Howard J. Rankin, Ph.D., behavioral psychology advisor for the TOPS (Take Off Pounds Sensibly) Club and author of *7 Steps to Wellness*. You have to determine a realistic rate of weight loss. A moderately active woman who eats 1,200 calories a day may lose only 3 pounds a month. So she needs to accept that it may take her almost a year to lose 30 pounds. "If you go to extremes to lose weight, the chances are high that you will put it all back on again when you return to a manageable lifestyle," Dr. Rankin says.

Anticipate obstacles. Determine how you're going to deal with potential problems like Thanksgiving, vacation, or a trip to McDonald's. "It's like going into war," says Dr. Haber. "You don't leave your weapons at home—you go to war prepared."

Break it down. Even a seemingly simple change involves a whole series of steps if it's to work. If you decide to munch carrots, celery, or bell peppers instead of chips while watching TV, make sure you went to the store to buy them. Then wash and peel them, cut them into sticks, and have ready a low-fat dip to make them taste good.

"There is a fair amount of energy and effort, particularly in the beginning of creating a new habit, that is very unnatural and requires a great deal of willpower," says Dr. Haber. Eventually, stashing a ready-to-eat supply of sliced fresh vegetables in your fridge will become second nature.

Enlist support. If possible, surround yourself with people who are supportive or join a support group like TOPS or Weight Watchers. "Overall, you really do need support if you're going to change your lifestyle," says Dr. Rankin. "It's an element of weight loss that is often overlooked." Support is a way of gathering information, getting encouragement, finding a facilitator, and keeping yourself anchored when you get off track.

Share your goals with friends and family. Show your spouse and other family members how they can help you, says Dr. Rankin. And keep in mind that some people in your life may actually hinder your efforts.

Action: Kick It into Gear

Stage 4: It's time to road test your plans.

You're psyched. But turning healthy eating and regular activity into lifelong habits requires determination and hard work.

Expect to encounter rough spots—situations where you're tempted to overeat and days when you'd rather have a root canal than break a sweat. To avoid quitting before you get to stage 5, you need to develop multiple strategies for dealing with everyday obstacles.

For instance, if you know that you tend to eat under stress, have a list of alternatives ready: a bubble bath, a glass of wine, a nap. Maybe write in your journal or call your best friend to rant. Keep the list posted on the refrigerator so it's the first thing you see when you reach for the cheesecake, suggests Dr. Marcus.

Remember these tips, too.

Give it time. New lifestyle habits aren't developed overnight. "You need time to focus on yourself and to practice your new eating and exercise habits," says Dr. Haber.

How much time differs for everyone, but generally 6 months of a new habit gives you enough time to build your confidence and your skills. By then, you'll have encountered your fair share of roadblocks—bad weather, travel, holidays—and found alternatives to stick with your new, healthy habits.

Make adjustments. Even if you've planned your strategy carefully, you may be struggling. Regularly reassess whether your program suits you and whether it makes you feel good, suggests Dr. Haber. This may mean revisiting stage 3. "The more you feel good about what you're doing, the more you'll look forward to it and keep it in your repertoire. The less you like it, the more quickly it's going to become a negative experience," she says.

Bask in the rewards. We frequently forget to congratulate ourselves for our small successes—walking every day for a week, passing on the dessert during a romantic dinner, achieving a 5-pound weight loss even if there are 15 more to go.

Also, pay attention to the benefits of eating better and leading a more active lifestyle, says Dr. Haber. If you have more energy, your clothes are fitting better, and people at work start commenting on how you look, it's a sure way to inspire yourself to stick with the program. And reward yourself occasionally. Buy a new piece of clothing, get a manicure, or go to a movie (but skip the buttered popcorn).

Be flexible. Slipping back into an all-or-nothing mode of thinking can trigger a relapse, says Dr. Marcus. Your plan to take a 1-hour walk at lunch evaporates when you get stuck taking a phone call. By the time you hang up, you have only 20 minutes to spare, so you figure the heck with it. Wrong, says Dr. Marcus. Some exercise is always better than none.

Maintenance: You've Got It Down

Stage 5: You're maintaining your new eating and exercise habits and are satisfied with the results.

If you've reached your weight-loss goal, give yourself a well-deserved shopping spree. But don't stop now. Use the skills you developed in earlier stages of change—focus on the benefits, reward yourself regularly, set goals, and vary your activities.

Mastering this stage requires patience and persistence and may take a year or more. A clue that you've truly progressed through all five stages of change: Your new lifestyle is automatic.

Expect to slip. Setbacks are a normal part of the process. Your biggest challenges may be times of emotional and psychological distress—when you're bored, stressed, angry, or lonely. Unfortunately, these are the times when many of us use food to cope. If you slip up for a day or two, says Dr. Haber, pick yourself up and get going again.

Learn to readjust. Suppose your job changes and you can no longer exercise when it's light out. Or your treadmill breaks. Don't let new barriers send you back a stage or two.

Be supportive. Share what you've learned with other women who are trying to lose weight, says Dr. Haber. Helping others reach their goals is a good way to remind yourself of how far you've come.

Excuses

When it comes to weight loss, we can whip out a page of excuses longer than our weekend to-do list. And whine? Man, we can put a 2-year-old to shame, whining about all the reasons "now is just not a good time" to change our lives, our weight, our eating habits.

Intellectually, we know all the reasons we should get on the weight-loss bandwagon: Our cholesterol is too high, we can't stand the way we look, we're always tired, and—oh, yeah—we'd like to live to see our grandkids. Emotionally, we just don't want to do it.

So we make excuses as to why we shouldn't even start; that way, we don't have to do the hard work.

Often, what we think of as excuses are really solvable obstacles, says Karen Miller-Kovach, R.D., chief scientist for Weight Watchers International. "Excuses are artificial," she says. "As soon as one is removed, another and another and another take its place. Whereas obstacles have solutions that can resolve the problem. The key is finding the solution that is acceptable to you. Otherwise, you won't keep at it for the long term."

And we're in this lifestyle change for, well, life.

With that in mind, here are some excuse busters from the experts—solid, simple-to-follow solutions that will dismantle your defenses and eradicate your excuses.

Excuse #1: Diets Don't Work for Me

That's true, and not just for you. It's true for everyone. Research proves what we instinctively know: Very little of the weight lost in diet programs is maintained over the long term.

"That's why you have to focus on lifestyle change," says Howard J. Rankin, Ph.D., behavioral psychology advisor for the TOPS (Take Off Pounds Sensibly) Club and author of *7 Steps to Wellness*.

Excuse Busters

Integrate exercise and healthy eating into your everyday life. "Don't view them as something you're going to do until you lose the weight, after which time you'll go back to your 'normal' life," says Dr. Rankin.

Stop viewing weight loss as something that should be done *for* you. "As in, diets don't work *for* me," says Kristi Ferguson, Ph.D., associate professor of community and behavioral health at the University of Iowa College of Public Health in Iowa City. "This is something you have to want to do for yourself."

Go to the doctor. In one study examining what motivated women to start losing weight, a strong trigger was their doctors' refusing to perform surgery unless the women lost weight or telling the women that their weight was making them sick.

Focus on the positives. Like more sex. In one study of 32 overweight women, more than half said that their sex lives improved after they lost weight. They thought about sex more, or had sex more often, because they felt better about their body image.

Excuse #2: My Metabolism Is Too Slow

"No matter how low your metabolism is, there's always something you can do to rev it up," says Dr. Rankin.

And forget the one about your metabolism slowing simply because of age. Some research indicates that most women put on about a pound a year between the ages of 30 and 40, not because of slowing metabolism but because of slowing up—eating more and moving less.

The less muscle mass you have, the slower your metabolism. And as you get older, you do have to work harder to maintain that muscle. Women lose about ½ pound of muscle a year during perimenopause and a pound a year during menopause. By age 55, if you're not increasing your activity level, that could equate to 15 pounds of muscle lost, meaning that you're burning 600 fewer calories per day.

Guilt-Free Pleasure: Aromatherapy

Scents affect your mood, says Barbara Close, president and founder of Naturopathica Holistic Health Spa in East Hampton, New York. Here's how aromatherapy can enhance your weight-loss efforts.

Choose your mood. If you have no energy when it's time for your daily walk, try a stimulating scent. Some examples: rosemary, peppermint, orange, grapefruit, and other citrus fruits.

Anxious, nervous—and ready to snack? Soothe yourself with the calming scents of lavender, sandalwood, vetiver, myrrh, and frankincense.

Excuse Busters

Lift weights. Weight-bearing exercise builds muscle, which burns up to 25 percent more calories all day long, even when you're sleeping.

Eat frequently. No, not Entenmann's and McDonald's. But frequently eating small, high-fiber, low-fat meals that include some protein can keep your metabolism humming, says Dr. Rankin. "Every time you eat, your metabolism goes up. In fact, about 15 percent of the calories eaten are quickly used up in the process of food digestion."

Push past the set points. The irony here is that as you lose weight, your metabolism really does decrease, making it harder for you to lose, says Dr. Ferguson.

Upping the intensity or length of your workout or changing the type of workout you're doing to challenge your body can give you a boost, says Tammy T. Baker, R.D., an Arizona-based spokesperson for the American Dietetic Association.

Insist on authentic. Buy 100 percent pure essential oils—extracted from the leaves and fruit of the plant—rather than synthetic. Natural scents are stronger.

Use scents creatively. Light scented candles, use a diffuser, or smooth scented lotion on your body. A couple of drops added to your humidifier will fill your room with scent for 2 hours. Mix several drops with an ounce of a carrier oil—almond, sunflower, or vegetable—and add it to your bath or give it to your significant other for a massage (never apply undiluted essential oils to your skin; they can burn you). And don't forget to scent your office with potpourri or oils.

Excuse #3: I Can't Afford to Join a Gym

So don't. They're expensive, loud, and filled with too many too-thin women in too-shiny spandex.

Excuse Busters

Work out at home. A University of Florida study of 49 women weighing an average of 190 pounds found that those who worked out at home lost more weight and did a better job of keeping it off than those who joined a group exercise program, like an aerobics class.

Swap. If you work out at home, you can replace the gym's Stairmaster with your teenager's bike, its treadmill with a pair of sneakers, and its weight machines with sets of lunges and crunches, followed by some lifting with a full water bottle in each hand.

Excuse #4: I'm Too Busy to Exercise

First of all, rid yourself of any preconceived notions about the word *exercise*. We're not talking a 45-minute run followed by a weight machine circuit.

We're talking movement, integrating more action into your daily life in ways that eventually will become so ingrained that you won't even realize you're doing them.

Simply increasing your normal activities of daily living—fidgeting, moving around, changing your posture—can help prevent weight gain even if your calorie intake doesn't change.

Excuse Busters

Turn off the TV. We watch an average of 22 hours of television a week. And every hour of TV can be blamed for an extra ½ pound of weight per year. Can't give up the tube for exercise? Put your stationary bike or treadmill in the family room, plopped right in front of the TV.

Build it into work. Let's start with e-mail. If you walk to someone's office for 2 minutes to deliver a message instead of spending 2 minutes at your desk typing an e-mail, you'll lose 1.1 pounds of fat a year. That's 11 pounds over a decade. Conversely, if you sit at your desk, you're going to *gain* that 11 pounds. This "creeping obesity" is associated with significant increases in blood pressure, cholesterol levels, and insulin resistance.

So get up. Go to the bathroom on a different floor. Never take the elevator (unless you're on the 43rd floor, in which case you can walk up at least 10 flights). Try pushups against your desk and stomach clenches while you're checking the aforementioned e-mail. Eventually, says Baker, you'll begin to see results.

Have a really clean house. We're talking the kind of clean that would satisfy even your mother-in-law. Vacuum every other day, including the furniture. Sweep the kitchen floor every night. Bend down and wipe those baseboards. Stretch up and clean the top of the refrigerator. And wear ankle weights while you're doing all this.

Pace while you're on the phone. Why do you think they invented the portable phone? You should do at least ¼ mile around the house for every 15-minute conversation, says Baker. A quarter mile would be about 40 return trips to the end of an average-size room and back. If your phone's not portable, get a long cord and pace as far as you can.

Act like a toddler. Watch how young children move, says Baker. They bounce around, climb the walls, and run from one room to the next with no purpose in mind. Ask them to bring you several things, and they're likely to bring them one at a time. "They're energy inefficient, and that's what it takes to burn calories," she says. You can do the same thing. Carry items upstairs one at a time. Eat dinner in the dining room so that you burn more calories setting the table, carrying the food in, and clearing up. And stop asking your kids to bring you things; go get them yourself.

Get it in short bursts. Three 10-minute bursts of exercise throughout the day are just as effective at burning calories as one 30-minute set, says Baker. (In fact, a 10-minute power walk burns 55 calories, and if you did just that once a day, you'd lose close to 6 pounds in a year.) Although you may not burn as many calories, you could break that 10 minutes down into even shorter increments. Waiting for the pasta water to boil? Drop and do 10 pushups. Waiting for the pasta to cook? Add a set of lunges.

Avoid drive-thrus. Park and walk into the bank, dry cleaner, or restaurant. Even standing in line burns more calories than sitting in your car.

Avoid machines. Instead of driving through the car wash, wash your car yourself (and wax it) to burn 306 calories in an hour. Use a rake instead of a leaf blower, a push mower instead of a powered one. Throw away the remote control and burn an extra 3 calories every time your show ends and you have to get up and change the channel.

Excuse #5: I Am Too Stressed to Make These Kinds of Changes

You just lost your job. You're in the midst of a divorce. You're moving into a new house. Maybe, you think, my life is too stressful.

Excuse Busters

Get real. "In reality, there's never going to be the ideal time to make these kinds of changes," says Dr. Rankin. "You can't expect life to stand still while you make changes."

Opt for a lifestyle change. Some studies show that it's not the major life traumas like divorce or losing your job that are most likely to result in physical symptoms but those annoying, everyday occurrences like car trouble or running late for work that drive us to the antacids and aspirin.

Why You Crave Chocolate

Simple: It makes you feel good.

When you're stressed, the sweet taste takes your mind off your problems. If you're hungry, candy raises your low blood sugar level. Premenstrual? You're craving carbohydrates, which help increase the levels of certain feel-good hormones in your brain.

Chocolate satisfies us more than other candies because of its mouth-watering combination of sugar and fat. And it's associated with good childhood memories: chocolate birthday cakes and heart-shaped Valentine's boxes. Maybe that's why chocolate soothes us more than apples when we're bored or stressed.

There would be nothing wrong with eating chocolate every day—if it weren't for our attitude problem. We know chocolate's full of fat, so we tell ourselves that we can't eat it. And whenever we deny ourselves something, we want it more. Before we know it, the whole box is gone.

But if you allow yourself one piece a day, you'll do just fine. A mini chocolate bar has 36 calories and 2 grams of fat. Add it to your daily meal plan and subtract that pat of butter on the baked potato. Maybe the "craving" for chocolate will stop and the enjoyment will start.

Expert consulted: Connie Diekman, R.D., spokesperson for the American Dietetic Association

Physical activity helps with that stress, and the activity doesn't have to be intense. In one study of 135 undergraduate university students, taking part in leisure-type physical activity like walking or riding a bike buffered the effects of stress more than intense aerobic activity like running.

Yet another study done by researchers at Duke University Medical Center in Durham, North Carolina, showed that the more physically fit a woman was—independent of regular exercise—the lower her blood pressure during a stressful day at work. This suggests that she's more able to remain calm during work-related stress.

Excuse #6: I Hate Cooking

"Cooking and good nutrition don't have to go hand in hand," says Baker. Nor does healthy eating mean that you can't use prepared or takeout foods as the cornerstone of your healthy diet.

Excuse Busters

Buy packaged meals. Even packaged dinners like Hamburger Helper or pasta salad mixes can be healthy. Cut in half the oil they call for (you'll never miss it), substitute soy burger crumbles or low-fat ground turkey for hamburger meat, and add in extra vegetables. In many cases, you can cut the calories by half and bring the fat down to nearly zero.

Do takeout. If Friday-night pizza is a staple at your house, don't change the routine, just the toppings. Instead of greasy pepperoni or sausage, order extra veggies and ask for half as much cheese on the pie. Or pick up a rotisserie-roasted chicken at the deli, then add pre-washed bagged salad and a 5-minute box of whole wheat couscous.

Buy prepared. More than half of us are buying those precut vegetables and prewashed salads. The reason? Convenience. So for a quick veggie to go with the takeout chicken, just dump some of those baby carrots into boiling water for 10 minutes and drain. Voilà! Instant vitamin A. It's healthy and it's easy—and that should be your meal mantra.

Try frozen. It takes most fruits and veggies a week or more to reach store shelves, and then they may sit for days or longer before they hit your dinner table, losing valuable vitamins in the process. Frozen vegetables, however, have as many vitamins and minerals as most fresh—and sometimes more because they're frozen immediately after harvesting.

Buy canned. Then there are the divine gifts to dinnertime: diced canned tomatoes and fat-free refried beans. Drain and spread those tomatoes on a prepared pizza shell, top with already shredded low-fat cheese, and call it dinner. Spread the refried beans on a whole wheat tortilla, add the same cheese and tomatoes, roll up, and microwave for 1 minute. Again, you've got a healthy, easy dinner that even your kids will eat.

Excuse #7: I Can't Afford Healthy Food

Nearly half of us think that fruits, vegetables, fish, and other "healthy" foods cost more than the frozen french fries and corn chips that we've been tossing into the shopping cart. Well, check the prices. "Studies show that the closer foods are to their natural form, like produce, the less expensive they are compared with the prepackaged stuff we buy," says Baker.

For example, investigators at Pennsylvania State University in State College and Mary Imogene Bassett Research Institute in Cooperstown, New York, gave 300 people with high cholesterol information on cutting fat from their diets. Those whose cholesterol levels dropped the most after 9 months had cut an average of $1.10 a day from their food bills—a yearly savings of $1,600 for a family of four. That's enough for a massage every month.

Excuse Busters

Shop smart. Buy produce in season. "It stands to reason that the strawberries shipped from Chile in January are

---

Are You Cranky When Hungry?

When you don't eat for several hours, your blood sugar level drops low enough to stress your body. As a result, you feel light-headed, you have trouble concentrating, you get sleepy—and you may get irritable.

Whether or not you get to the cranky stage depends on how long since you ate and what you had. You don't need to eat while you're sleeping, but you need to replenish your fuel stores constantly during the day. You should eat 3 to 5 hours after meals and 2 to 3 hours after a snack. Grabbing a piece of hard candy or a can of soda doesn't do it—these simple carbohydrates cause your blood sugar to spike, but it's a temporary rise. Just as quickly, it plunges, leaving you even hungrier, shakier, and more irritable.

To avoid those irritable feelings, eat some protein—like lean turkey or beans—with every meal. Protein is digested more slowly, keeping your blood sugar level and your mood on a more even keel.

Expert consulted: Claudia Plaisted, R.D., director of the nutrition and medicine program, University of North Carolina, Chapel Hill

going to cost more than the strawberries grown in the farm outside of town in May," says Baker.

Save more than just calories. Eating healthy can pad your wallet. You won't be buying high-calorie fast food and greasy snacks out of vending machines. "Plus, if you're healthy, you're more productive, and you have fewer medical bills," says Dr. Rankin. Not to mention the money saved on antacids and aspirin.

Excuse #8: I Hate Fruits and Vegetables

Oh, really? When's the last time you passed on the carrot cake or refused that double scoop of strawberry ice cream?

Eating fruits and vegetables doesn't have to mean substituting an apple for a piece of chocolate cake. Although raw fruits and veggies do pack the greatest amount of fiber and nutrients, nutritionists are happy if you get them any way you can.

Excuse Busters

Hide them. Try smoothies made with fruit, low-fat milk, and fat-free yogurt. Grate carrots into spaghetti sauce. Puree apples and pears with a pinch of sugar to make luscious sauces for pork, chicken, or fish.

Don't ignore the obvious. Onions count. So does the garlic in your pasta sauce, the celery in your tuna salad, and the can of tomato juice you drank as a midmorning snack. And what about that salsa you ate with your corn chips?

Go for sweet. Substitute dried fruit for candy. Just 2 tablespoons count as one fruit serving. Try dried cranberries, papaya, or cherries.

Puree them. Add them to soups, stews, and sauces. A word of warning, says Baker: Don't mix different-colored vegetables together if the sauce is supposed to add color to the dish. You'll end up with an unappetizing brown mess.

Excuse #9: I Absolutely Cannot Live without My Ice Cream (Potato Chips, French Fries, Etc.)

So don't. There should be no four-letter words used here (like d-e-n-y). "Just eat less of it, but don't give it up entirely," says Dr. Ferguson.

Excuse Busters

Try low-fat. But be careful. Don't double the quantity just because the fat is gone, says Baker. Low-fat isn't necessarily low-calorie, and it is calories that count in weight loss.

Try portion control. The minute you bring the grocery bags in, portion out your treats into manageable amounts. Scoop ice cream into single-serving containers and freeze. Divvy up potato chips into individual storage bags. Wrap cookies two at a time in foil and store in your pantry.

Excuse #10: I Eat Out Too Much

Hey, even McDonald's understands that some of us are trying to eat healthfully. That's why most fast-food restaurants have numerous selections that are relatively harmless in terms of fat and calories, like plain hamburgers (270 calories), salads with fat-free dressing (85 calories), and grilled chicken sandwiches (300 calories).

Excuse Busters

Order light. Restaurants now have to abide by strict government rules when they call something light. For example, low-fat foods can't have more than 3 grams of fat per standard serving. Menus must disclose why a light (or "lite") food is called that. Is it the color, taste, or calories? But be careful on the serving sizes. Most restaurant portions are two to three times the standard, meaning two to three times the calories.

Know your restaurants. Particularly if you tend to eat lunch out every day, become familiar with restaurants around your office, then pick two or three healthy options at each. When you go, don't even look at the menu, with its tempting descriptions and high-calorie, high-fat options. Just order your already chosen selection.

Taste your food. Not sure if something is fat-filled? Pay attention to how it feels in your mouth. If it coats your teeth and the back of your mouth or if it makes your lips feel slippery, chances are it's fattening.

Excuse #11: My Family Won't Eat the Healthy Stuff

Heard the one about the couple who were eating a low-fat, nutritionally healthy diet? Only one of them knew it.

That's because there are many changes that you can sneak into your family's meals so gradually that by the time you tell them the steak and mashed potato dinner you just fixed is healthy, they'll think you've finally lost it. But they won't know that you chose the leanest cut of beef, cooked it so the fat drained off, used chicken broth instead of butter in the mashed potatoes, made that salsa with four different kinds of vegetables, and substituted applesauce for the vegetable oil in the dessert brownies.

Excuse Busters

Control portions. If your husband must have meat every night, then give him meat every night. But choose lean cuts of beef, poultry, and pork, and trim off every visible piece of fat. He may get 10 ounces. You should take only a 3-ounce serving, about the size of a deck of cards.

Add food. "You can generally sneak in one healthy food that you like at each meal," says Baker. "Make a lot of it so that you can eat a lot of it."

Watch the nibbles. "An awful lot of calories get consumed when you're preparing or cleaning up from a meal," Baker says. Before doing either, brush your teeth or chew a stick of gum. These steps will take away your taste for crumbs and leftovers.

Excuse #12: I'm around My Kids (and Their Food) All Day

You have the hardest job in the world: You're a stay-at-home mom. And that means fetching 10,000 cups of juice a day, making 400 peanut butter and jelly sandwiches, and handing out at least 200 Popsicles (more or less). And of course, kids never eat everything on their plates. That's where you come in.

Excuse Busters

Stop eating like a mom. This means throwing away the extra three chicken nuggets they didn't eat, scraping the ½ cup of macaroni and cheese into the garbage, and keeping your hands out of the Halloween candy.

Stop eating like a kid. If you're fixing them hot dogs and potato chips with sliced apples for lunch, fix yourself a lean turkey sandwich on whole wheat bread with lettuce and tomato, throw in some carrot sticks, and share the apples. If they're having plain pasta with butter for dinner, make yours with just a sprinkle of olive oil and load it up with steamed veggies.

Excuse #13: I Can Never Remember How Much I've Eaten during the Day

Given the warp speed at which you run your life, you're lucky you can remember your ATM password. Remember what you ate that morning? Please . . .

Excuse Busters

Write it down. In one study, those who were most consistent about writing down what they ate lost an average of 7 more pounds during the 6-week period between Thanksgiving and New Year's (the Bermuda triangle of weight loss) than those who didn't. In fact, those who didn't use a food diary ended up gaining 3 pounds.

Stock up. If you stock your pantry and fridge with only healthy foods—vegetables, fruits, beans, lean protein, whole wheat grains—you won't have to worry so much about portions. Eat until you feel full.

Excuse #14: I Need to Lose So Much Weight, There's No Point in Even Starting

The weight you need to lose looms before you like a mountain. It's easier, you think, to just walk around it than try to scale it. But consider this: Even a mountain climber starts with just one step.

Excuse Buster

Start small. One pound at a time—that's how you put it on, and that's how you'll take it off and keep it off.

Excuse #15: I Just Had a Baby

When you look at yourself in a full-length mirror, you don't see much difference between your reflection and a

She Feels Better than at 25

Twenty-five years ago, Peggy Malecha, a TOPS area captain for Arizona, weighed 225 pounds. Then her father died from vascular problems related to obesity, and her mother died from complications of diabetes. So she vowed to start exercising.

Unfortunately, she hated exercising. She had a list of excuses, from lack of time to hurting knees. How did she get herself moving? She added activity into her week slowly, instead of jumping into an intense exercise routine.

She started out with low-impact aerobics twice a week. Gradually, she increased to three times a week, combining aerobics with walking. Finally, she joined a gym, where she began weight training and high-impact aerobics. With the strength training, she helped her knees by strengthening

woman in her sixth month. All the more reason to get the weight off. But you can barely get yourself dressed by 5:00 P.M., let alone find time for a diet and exercise. Besides, you're up all night with the baby. Who has the energy?

Excuse Busters

If you already are breastfeeding, continue to do so. Numerous studies show that it's best for the baby: breastfed babies have fewer ear infections and allergies and optimal growth and development. But it's also great for you. You'll burn an extra 500 calories a day just feeding the baby, and you have an enormous incentive to eat healthy, says Baker. But don't expect miracles. "Your body does hold on to fat when estrogen levels are high," she says, as they are in nursing mothers and mothers of newborns.

her leg muscles. She realized that the more often she went, the more she enjoyed exercising and the less often those excuses slipped from her lips. Soon, exercising wasn't torture.

"Each time I lift a heavier weight and do aerobics a bit longer, it gives me a high," she says. "I finally made up my mind that I wasn't going to be a fat person again. Like an alcoholic who can't drink anymore, I'm an obese person who can't overeat anymore. The biggest benefit of exercise is being able to maintain my weight while eating a lot of healthy food."

Today, she bench-presses 50 pounds, leg-presses 180 pounds, has more stamina than she did at 25, and doesn't feel any more pain in her knees.

Leave the house. Once life has settled down a bit and you're getting at least 4 consecutive hours of sleep, there's nothing better than putting baby in a stroller and taking you both for a walk, says Baker. "It's good for the baby to get out of the house and see new things and have new learning experiences."

A study at the University of Michigan in Ann Arbor suggests that if you exercise, you'll not only wind up retaining less baby weight but also feel better about yourself overall and be more likely to do other fun things—like visit friends and family, pursue your hobbies, or go to the movies—than women who don't exercise.

Too cold or rainy to walk outside? Head for the mall. But leave the credit cards at home!

Excuse #16: I Just Quit Smoking

This is going to be tough, no doubt about it, says Miller-Kovach, since smoking typically consumes about 100 calories a day. But knowing this, you can resolve to eat 100 fewer calories a day or walk an extra mile per day (which consumes 100 calories).

Excuse Buster

Exercise will help you stay smoke-free. A study at Brown University in Providence, Rhode Island, of 281 women showed that vigorous exercise actually helped them quit and stay smoke-free more easily and longer than women who didn't exercise. The reason, the authors speculate, is that physical activity not only limits weight gain but also helps us better handle stress.

Weight-Loss Myths

Every day seems to bring some brand-new theory about what's to blame for weight gain. One day, it's genetics. The next, it's sugar and fat. Later, we hear that we should be eating nothing but protein or maybe only carbohydrates.

If you're left confused—and frustrated—by all the contradictory information, join the crowd.

The reality is that much of the diet news we get is based on unproven scientific evidence. "Women should focus less on these news stories and much more on what they're eating and how much they're exercising on a daily basis," says Judith Wurtman, Ph.D., a nutrition research scientist at the Massachusetts Institute of Technology in Cambridge.

"Many diet myths are simply made-up theories that make it seem as though everyone is overweight for the same reasons. But we're not," says Denise Bruner, M.D., president of the American Society of Bariatric Physicians (a group of doctors who specialize in weight-loss treatments) and a physician practicing in Arlington, Virginia.

Some women are heavy because they nibble all day long. Others overeat only at mealtimes. Many never exercise. And some have true eating disorders, says Dr. Bruner. All these factors must be handled differently. "Weight gain isn't all about eating too much of any one particular food or substance," she says.

Here's the straight scoop on many common weight-loss beliefs.

Myth #1: It's All in My Genes

The tendency toward large hips and thighs does run in families. And animal studies show that fat genes can affect how much we eat, our daily activity levels, and the speed of our metabolisms. An unlucky few are born with slower metabolisms than the rest of the world, but that's pretty rare.

"We've also learned that there are so many different fat genes that it would be impossible for people not to have at least some of them," says Teresa M. Gunn, Ph.D., a molecular genetics researcher at the Howard Hughes Medical Institute at Stanford University Medical Center.

But that doesn't necessarily mean you're doomed to be fat. In fact, only 40 percent of obesity is hereditary. The remaining 60 percent is a direct result of what you eat and how much physical activity you get.

And while the number of obese Americans has risen dramatically over the past 20 years, with more than 50 percent of the population now considered overweight, we can't blame it on our genes because the gene pool doesn't change that quickly, says Suzanne W. Dixon, R.D., a research epidemiologist and registered dietitian at the Henry Ford Health System in Detroit.

What may be to blame is our lifestyle. We live in a

high-tech society that keeps us sitting on our behinds in front of computer screens. We have drive-thru banking, grocery delivery, automatic garage door openers, and Internet shopping. Rather than cook healthy meals, we

Eat Up—And Lose Weight

Relax. You don't have to eat foods you hate in order to lose weight. You needn't live on cottage cheese or give up roast pork and buttery mashed potatoes.

Just identify the foods you absolutely can't live without and try to fit them into your diet plan. You can modify your recipes to make them less fattening (lots of magazines and cookbooks do that for you). Or you can eat your favorite foods as they are, but only in small quantities and on special occasions.

A clever way to incorporate the lower-fat, healthier foods you don't really like is to make them part of a larger recipe. For instance, make cream of broccoli soup that calls for yogurt as an ingredient. Eat cottage cheese with your favorite fruit. Try Chinese vegetable dishes instead of the veggies you grew up on.

If you want red meat, nix the burger or steak and opt for beef-vegetable soup, beef stir-fry, or a beef stew loaded with carrots, broccoli, and potatoes. That way, you scale back on the amount of meat you're eating while getting the vegetables you need.

Try to look at your weight-loss goals as opportunities to experiment with low-fat, healthy foods such as Japanese noodle dishes or Thai and Vietnamese cuisine. Chances are you'll love these new choices and won't feel deprived.

Expert consulted: Judith Wurtman, Ph.D., nutrition research scientist, Massachusetts Institute of Technology, Cambridge

order in. Then there are the ever-present vending machines and fast-food restaurants.

We're simply taking in too many calories and burning too few of them, says Dr. Bruner.

Myth #2: I've Reached My Set Point

Some experts believe that we're programmed from birth to be a certain size. This is known as the set-point theory. According to this theory, our brains program our metabolisms to speed up or slow down to maintain a set body weight, and there is nothing we can do to change that,

Stay Slim after 40

Once you hit your forties, it's definitely easier to pack on the pounds than it is to take them off. Your chances of weight gain increase as your metabolism slows, your hormones go haywire, and your stress level soars.

Solutions? First, set aside time for daily exercise. Ideally, you should get at least 30 minutes of cardiovascular activity followed by light weight training. Brisk walking, jogging, cycling, or step aerobics crank up your metabolism so that you burn fat and calories. Weight training boosts fat-burning power because it builds muscle mass. The more muscle you have, the more calories you burn— day and night. For every pound of muscle gained, you burn an extra 35 to 50 calories a day.

If you don't weight train, you'll lose about 7 to 10 pounds of muscle every 10 years after age 40. That's 350 fewer calories a day that you'll burn than you did when you were in your twenties.

says Dixon. So if we overeat, we burn more calories than usual, and if we eat less through dieting, our bodies burn fewer calories. This would mean a lucky few will stay slender no matter how much they eat. And others will hold on to those extra pounds no matter how little they consume.

But while many experts acknowledge that metabolism varies among different people, there's actually no strong scientific evidence proving that the set point exists.

"The idea that we're destined to be a certain weight is hotly debated by scientists," says Donna Ryan, M.D., an endocrinologist at Pennington Center in Baton Rouge,

Although you can't do much to control your hormones, you can take a bite out of stress. Studies show that chronic stress causes your body to produce high levels of the hormone cortisol, which weakens your immune system and deposits fat deep inside your belly. That type of fat is implicated as a cause in diabetes, high blood pressure, heart disease, stroke, and possibly cancer.

The best stress relievers are aerobic exercise, weight training, yoga, meditation, and socializing. The key is to minimize the stressors in your life and insist on making time for yourself. If your job is a problem, find one that's less demanding. If it's your husband and family, get help. That way, you won't feel so overwhelmed, and you'll avoid jeopardizing your health.

Expert consulted: Pamela Peeke, M.D., assistant clinical professor of medicine, University of Maryland, Bethesda, and author of *Fight Fat after Forty*

Louisiana. "Americans are fatter than ever before, yet we have the same genes."

Weight-loss experts are exploring the possibility that we may instead have a "settling point." In other words, once we reach a certain weight, our bodies want to stay right where they are, no matter what. That would explain why 60 percent of successful weight losers regain every pound within 2 years, and 90 percent gain the weight back within 5 years, says Dr. Ryan. So some people, because of their metabolism, may have to work a little harder at monitoring what they eat and maintaining their physical activity in order not to regain the weight.

Myth #3: Food Is Addictive

Food is the centerpiece at family gatherings, office meetings, and parties. And it's a necessity we can't live without. So in a sense, aren't we all food addicts?

Not really. Food addiction is defined as an unhealthy preoccupation with food and an inability to stop eating a particular food. It can take the form of emotional eating due to depression, anger, boredom, frustration, or exhaustion. And it can show itself as a compulsive eating disorder like bulimia or anorexia nervosa.

Some women use food for other reasons, such as a coping mechanism for dealing with stress. These women often have underlying psychological issues that they're not addressing, such as boredom, loneliness, and low self-esteem, says Dixon. "They need to address them if their food dependence is going to be resolved."

Myth #4: Diets Are the Best Way to Lose Weight

Extreme dieting is one of the worst things you can do. When you cut way back on calories, you rob your body of vital nutrients. That sets off a complex chain of events that eventually slams the brakes on your metabolism. If you don't eat, your body thinks you're starving. So your fat-burning engines cool down and hang on to what fuel you have left. You may lose weight initially, but the pounds become harder to drop as time goes on, in part because of nutritional deficiencies.

Here's the real kicker: Once you start eating again, it may take a while for your engine to heat back up. As a result, you may gain back the pounds you lost—and then some. "If you've been yo-yo dieting all of your life, chances are your metabolism is at its slowest," says Dr. Bruner. "It's your body's way of protecting itself from starving to death."

Diets can also put you in a constant state of deprivation, which can lead to bingeing on high-fat foods. "The critical mistake dieters make is that they eat very small portions and skip meals," says Dr. Ryan. "They'll forgo breakfast, drink a diet soda for lunch, and eat a low-calorie microwave dinner. They're starving. And when they do start eating again, they can't stop. So bingeing is really a physiological response to starvation."

Myth #5: I Need to Reduce Portion Sizes

Downsizing portion sizes at mealtimes can help you lose weight initially, but if you don't add regular exercise to the equation, you won't keep the pounds off. Why? Because there will always be days when you eat a few extra cookies or potato chips. The exercise will burn those excess calories to help you maintain your figure, says Dr. Bruner.

Myth #6: Fat Makes Me Fat

Fat packs 9 calories per gram, compared with 4 in carbohydrates and protein, so it can do the most damage to your figure if you eat too much of it. "But losing weight isn't just about calculating grams of fat. It's about counting calories," says Dixon.

"There was a time when you could reduce your fat intake and lose weight, but with all the high-calorie processed foods now available, you often end up eating even more calories that get stored as fat," says Dr. Ryan.

Myth #7: I Can Eat All the Carbohydrates I Want

Gram for gram, carbohydrates are lower in calories than fat. Vegetables, whole grains, and beans are great sources of complex carbohydrates, while most cereals, cookies, and soda provide the simple carbs that we sometimes call sugars. Other foods, such as fruits and potatoes, fall somewhere in the middle because they contain both complex and simple carbohydrates. People forget that if you concentrate on complex carbohydrates, you end up eating fewer calories. As a bonus, the fiber contained in complex carbohydrates helps fill you up and keeps you full longer than simple carbohydrates, so you eat less.

So, on one level, carbohydrates really are good for you. The problem is, ever since fat was labeled as the enemy, people have been loading up on simple carbohydrates, not realizing that they were eating more food and exceeding the number of calories they needed, says Dixon. "And if your body isn't using these simple carbohydrates, they turn to fat," says Dr. Bruner.

Myth #8: Alcohol Is No Problem

Some studies show that alcohol causes weight gain; others suggest it doesn't, says Dr. Bruner.

But the reality is that your body doesn't distinguish between the calories from alcohol and those from food, says Dr. Wurtman. If your body doesn't use the calories from alcohol as energy, it will convert them into fat. Also, some research shows that alcohol drinking can actually lead to overeating. One reason is that when we drink, our willpower isn't as strong, so we may give in to the temptation to overeat. If you're trying to drop a few pounds, it's wise to put down the wineglass, says Dr. Wurtman.

Realities

At Boston's Fenway Park, what people complain about most is not the antiquated restrooms or lack of skyboxes but the cramped seats. In a brand-new stadium planned for the city, fans will ease into bigger aisles and wider, comfier seating.

Detroit remedied a similar problem when it built its new Comerica Park and installed molded plastic seats that are 2 inches wider than the 17-inch wooden ones in the old Tiger Stadium.

What used to be regular size just doesn't fit our expanding proportions anymore. More than half of us are overweight these days, according to the Centers for Disease Control and Prevention. And the problem is getting worse every year. Between 1991 and 1998, the proportion of Americans who were obese (more than 30 percent above their ideal body weight) increased by 50 percent. Why?

What Will Be Will Be

Traditionally, society has blamed fatness on the individual. We assume that we're overweight because of our own personal failings—we're undisciplined, lazy, gluttonous, and lacking in willpower. Well, guess what. Some of the factors that contribute to our being overweight are clearly out of our control. For example:

Genes. A family history of obesity increases your chances of becoming obese by about 25 to 30 percent. But heredity isn't destiny—your genes alone cannot make you overweight, says Michele L. Trankina, Ph.D., professor of biological sciences at St. Mary's University of San Antonio and a nutritional consultant. What they can do is make you more susceptible to gaining weight by influencing metabolism, body type, appetite, and even how active you are from moment to moment—in other words, how much you fidget.

Tempting as it may be to blame your DNA, remember that it's only a small part of the equation.

Age. With age come wisdom, laugh lines, and a few more pounds. "It's not a matter of *if* we'll gain but when and how much," says Linda Van Horn, R.D., Ph.D., professor in the department of preventive medicine at Northwestern University Medical School in Chicago. Research shows that on average women gain about a pound a year between ages 30 and 40. By the time the average woman settles into her forties, there's a 30 percent chance she weighs too much. And it doesn't stop there. The pounds continue to pile on. By the time women pass menopause, more than half are overweight.

The explanation is simple. As we age, we burn fewer calories, says Miriam Nelson, Ph.D., associate chief of the Human Physiology Laboratory at the Jean Mayer USDA Human Nutrition Research Center on Aging at Tufts University in Boston and author of *Strong Women Stay Slim*. The basal metabolic rate of an average 60-year-old is 200 calories lower than that of a 30-year-old woman. Most of that metabolic slowdown can be explained by a loss of muscle mass due to a sedentary lifestyle.

Each pound of muscle burns from 35 to 50 calories a day; fat burns a measly 2 calories. Starting around age 40, most women lose about ⅓ pound of muscle a year and add at least that much fat, explains Dr. Nelson. With the approach of menopause, these changes in body composition speed up. If you lose 5 pounds of muscle, you burn up to 250 fewer calories a day.

Gender. Women are genetically endowed with more body fat and slower metabolisms than men. So it's easier for us to gain weight. "A woman's fat cells are physio-

A Tale of Two Lifestyles

In the Gila River Indian Community in Arizona, it's not unusual for a kindergartner to weigh 75 pounds. Or for an adult to weigh 300 pounds. More than two-thirds of the 11,000 Pima Indians who live there are obese, and half the adults have diabetes.

Their genes are partly to blame. Like other Native Americans, the Pimas may possess a "thrifty gene" that encourages energy storage during times of plenty to tide them over in times of famine. But there's more to the story.

The Pimas settled as farmers in the Southwest nearly 2,000 years ago, establishing a sophisticated irrigation system in the desert that helped them produce wheat, beans, squash, and cotton. Their lives were active, while their diets were high in fiber and very low in fat.

Life changed drastically in 1890, when their water supply was diverted by European settlers. Starving and no longer able to farm, the Pima community had to rely on food provided by the federal government—mostly lard,

logically different from a man's. They are larger, more active, and more resistant to dieting," says Debra Waterhouse, R.D., author of *Outsmarting the Midlife Fat Cell.*

Time of life. There are certain points in our lives where we're *programmed* to gain weight.

"The average woman has 30 billion fat cells," says Waterhouse. During puberty, pregnancy, and menopause, fat cells respond to increased or decreased estrogen levels by expanding and multiplying. So we typically get fatter during the major hormonal shifts that occur with these life-altering events.

sugar, and white flour. Today sedentary office jobs predominate, and fatty, processed foods are the norm.

There's a second, small Pima community in Mexico's Sierra Madre. Their ancestors separated from the main tribe nearly 1,000 years ago. On average, they are nearly 60 pounds lighter than their American cousins and six times less likely to develop diabetes.

The Mexican Pimas spend 23 hours a week in hard physical exercise, while the Arizonans spend less than 5. There are no laborsaving devices, not even electricity. They eat a traditional diet of fruits, vegetables, beans, and tortillas, all of which are high in fiber and low in animal fat.

For scientists, the striking physical difference between the two branches of the Pimas perfectly illustrates the impact of modern living on weight and health.

"Here's strong evidence that lifestyle can win out over genetics," says Leslie Schulz, Ph.D., professor of health sciences at the University of Wisconsin–Madison.

A female's fat cells also start acting a little more male during midlife. Instead of attaching themselves to our hips and thighs, they accumulate around the abdomen.

Society. Simply living in America in the 21st century puts us at risk for weight gain, says Marion Nestle, Ph.D., professor and chairperson of the department of nutrition and food studies at New York University in New York City. We have access to a cornucopia of high-fat, high-calorie, good-tasting foods that are widely available, low in cost, and heavily promoted. "Food is an $800 billion industry in this country, and the objective of the food industry is to encourage people to eat more food, not less," says Dr. Nestle. The fact is, in our culture it's getting awfully hard *not* to be fat.

Consider these facts:

- Between 1970 and 1993, some 2,500 kinds of candy, gum, and snacks entered the market. During the same time period, about 1,500 new kinds of baked goods were introduced.
- Eight percent of Americans eat at McDonald's on any given day. The corporate goal is to have no American more than 4 minutes from one of its restaurants. And that's only one fast-food chain.
- The average American child sees 20,000 advertisements a year on television, and fast-food and food-product ads are ranked as the favorite among kids, so the food industry is obviously getting their attention.

But all this talk about food ignores the other side of the equation. Most of us are bulging not just because we consume too many calories but because we burn too few. From the electric can opener to the garage door opener, labor-saving devices have necessitated the need for increased exercise in order to stay slim.

Weight-loss experts are acknowledging the link between the environment in which we now live and how much weight we've gained in the past decade. It's unlikely that these changes are caused by lack of motivation or genetic or other biological changes in the population.

The Risk Factors You Control

In one survey, doctors and scientists involved in obesity research were asked to name the most important cause of weight gain. Their answer: genetics, a risk factor we can't control. In another study, researchers at Wesleyan University in Middletown, Connecticut, asked the same ques-

Massage: More than Pure Pampering

A massage is a good way to feel more positive about your body image, even before you lose weight. "Women often tell me they were apprehensive about coming in for a massage because they are overweight," says Mary Beth Packard, a registered massage therapist practicing in Fort Worth, Texas. "But after one session, they're completely comfortable with it. Massage is a good way to get back in touch with your body."

Massage also offers physical and psychological bonuses. The long, smooth strokes against the skin improve circulation and soothe the nervous system, explains Packard. The result: relief of muscle tension and stress. And stress, as we all know, can quickly sabotage any attempt at weight loss. "Massage is a good way to calm things down so that you may be less likely to overeat," she says.

Don't be surprised if you also notice that your skin glows and your digestion improves—two more key benefits of massage.

tion of 3,400 people who actually were obese. They got some very different answers.

Both women and men believed that lack of exercise and enjoyment of eating were the most important reasons for their weight gain. "This was encouraging," says Ruth Striegel-Moore, Ph.D., professor of psychology at Wesleyan University and coauthor of the study, "because it showed that overweight people were focusing on aspects of their lifestyle that they could change."

Regardless of our genes, age, or gender, the biggest risk factors involved in weight gain are lifestyle choices that we can control.

Here are some ways to take control of them in your own life.

Make muscles. Maintaining muscle is the single most important thing you can do to rev your metabolism and avoid middle-age spread, says Barbara Moore, Ph.D., president of Shape Up America! in Washington, D.C. Challenging your muscles for as little as 20 to 30 minutes twice a week with regular strength training can do the trick.

"We can increase our basal metabolic rates by 15 percent or more simply by building muscle," says Dr. Nelson. One thing you need to be aware of is that your basal metabolic rate, or BMR (the number of calories you burn at rest), is responsible for about 75 percent of the calories you burn. And the single most important factor in determining BMR is how much lean tissue you have in your body.

Fill up with fiber. When you reach for the cookies instead of the fruit, or the pretzel sticks instead of the carrot sticks, you're missing out on fiber. And a high-fiber diet may fight weight gain, according to a 10-year study of more than 2,900 young adults. Participants who ate at least 21 grams of fiber a day gained 8 fewer pounds on average over the 10-year period than people who ate the least fiber.

"Fiber helps regulate appetite by making you feel full," says Dr. Van Horn, a coauthor of the study. It also speeds food through your system so that you absorb fewer calories.

Once known as roughage, fiber is found only in plant foods—fruits, vegetables, whole grains, legumes (beans, peas, and lentils), nuts, and seeds. It's the part of the plant that you don't digest. The average American woman consumes fewer than half of the 25 to 30 grams that experts recommend.

Make time for you. Too busy to chop fresh vegetables, cook a healthy meal, or take a walk? Maybe it's because you put your needs after everyone else's. "The biggest excuse I hear is 'I don't have time.' I call it the type E personality—everything for everybody," says Dr. Trankina. "By the time we take care of everyone else, we're exhausted." The daily time crunch is at the root of a lot of the risky behaviors that contribute to weight gain, from skipping meals to eating whatever's handy or sitting on the couch instead of stepping on the Stairmaster.

Focus on calories, not fat. "We think that by cutting fat, we can ignore calories," says Dr. Moore. Consumption of fat declined from 37 percent of total calories in 1965 to 34 percent in 1991. At the same time, our calorie intake has climbed from 1,989 to 2,153 per day.

Low-fat often doesn't equal low-cal. A fat-free fig cookie has only 10 fewer calories than the original version. Two tablespoons of low-fat peanut butter give you only 10 fewer calories than the full-fat version.

But it doesn't end there. When our eyes see "low-fat," our brains say "eat more." To test how "low-fat" and "fat-free" labels affect food intake, researchers at Pennsylvania State University in University Park gave 48 women three indistinguishable raspberry-flavored yogurts. When the women ate the yogurts labeled "low-fat," they consumed significantly more calories during the subsequent lunch and dinner than they did after eating the yogurt labeled "high-fat." When the yogurts weren't labeled for fat content, these differences didn't occur.

You Are What You Drink

You may gain weight because of what you drink, not what you eat. Researchers at Purdue University in West Lafayette, Indiana, found that when people consume solid foods, they compensate for those calories by eating less of other foods. When they consume beverages, however, total calorie intake goes up, and so does their weight.

Americans are drinking more caloric beverages than ever. Since the 1970s, soda consumption has more than doubled. We're drinking more soda than coffee, tea, and juice combined. This averages out to about 56 gallons of the sugary stuff per person per year—a mind-boggling 85,263 calories a year.

Skip the soda and opt for eight 8-ounce glasses of water a day, says Denise Bruner, M.D., president of the American Society of Bariatric Physicians and a physician practicing in Arlington, Virginia. Besides having zero calories, water fills you up so you eat less. It also helps your body metabolize stored fat and clear your system of wastes.

Dr. Bruner has her patients fill a bottle with their daily water allotment and keep it on their desks at work or on the kitchen table at home. "Make a pact with yourself that you're not going home until you finish those cups," she says.

Move it all around. Nearly two-thirds of us get less than 2½ hours of activity each week. Whether we're sitting behind the wheel or parked in front of the television, physical inactivity is now built into our lives the same way strenuous labor was a natural part of daily life for our ancestors.

Today the average woman expends about half the energy that her great-grandmother did each day. Our sedentary lifestyle is one of the main reasons we're seeing a steady rise in the obesity rate, say a number of experts.

"We now know that most women aren't getting heavier because they eat more," says Dr. Nelson. "The surprising reason many women gain weight is that they burn too few calories."

Ditch the diets. One out of every four Americans is currently dieting, according to the Calorie Control Council. Most middle-age women have been on at least 15 diets since their teenage years. You'd think that with all this dieting we'd be getting thin. But we aren't, because diets are fattening.

Diets boost the ability of our fat cells to store fat, to take in new fat, and sometimes to multiply even further, says Waterhouse. Fat cells evolved to take care of us during times of famine—or calorie restriction—by holding on to the fat we have and becoming more aggressive at taking in new fat once the diet is over.

What's more, rationing your calories too stringently triggers hormonal shifts that help your body conserve calories instead of burning them. And at least 25 to 30 percent of the weight you lose by dieting is water, muscle, bone, and other lean tissue—not fat. The faster you lose weight, the more lean tissue you lose.

All of this points to a slower metabolism. In fact, the

wrong diet can reduce your metabolic rate by up to 30 percent.

Eat where you sleep. The increase in obesity closely follows the trend of eating away from home more often, says Dr. Nestle. "The more we eat out, the more we eat, and the fatter we get."

It's no wonder. A typical restaurant meal *without* an appetizer or dessert contains 1,000 calories. A study of 129 people found that those who ate out the most—more than six times per week—consumed an average of 300 more calories a day than people who ate out less often. The extra calories, which came primarily from fat, didn't add up to extra nutrition either, notes Linda Eck Clemens, R.D., Ed.D., professor of clinical nutrition at the University of Memphis, who led the study.

Think small. When was the last time your family got seven servings from a 7-ounce bag of chips? From supersize fast-food fries to a movie theater box of chocolates, we tend to eat more when we buy large sizes, says Dr. Nestle. People often eat 25 to 50 percent more—especially pure-pleasure foods like candy, chips, and buttered popcorn—when these foods come in bigger sizes.

"We buy large sizes because we perceive them as a good value," says Dr. Nestle. But we've lost our sense of exactly how big one portion should be. One hundred students taking a nutrition course were asked to bring in a bagel, baked potato, muffin, or cookie that they considered "medium." Then they compared those foods with the serving sizes that the USDA considers medium. Here are the results.

- A typical medium baked potato was 7 ounces, instead of the USDA's 4 ounces.
- A typical medium bagel was 4 ounces, double the USDA's 2 ounces.

- A typical medium muffin was 6 ounces, triple the USDA's 2 ounces.

It's not enough to make smart choices about what you're eating. You also have to pay attention to how much.

Write it down. When it comes to remembering what we've eaten during the day, a lot of us develop a case of food amnesia. So keeping a food journal can be helpful. "We get busy and tend to forget what we've eaten," says Denise Bruner, M.D., president of the American Society of Bariatric Physicians and a physician practicing in Arlington, Virginia. And without an awareness of what you've actually consumed, the calories can add up before you can say double cheeseburger.

Following Fads

Alice isn't stashing pretzels in her pantry anymore—or anything else that's low-fat, for that matter. In fact, so far today, she has eaten steak and eggs for breakfast, pork rinds for a snack, sliced ham for lunch, more pork rinds in the afternoon, ground beef patties for dinner. Now she stares at that bag of shriveled, gnarly strips of pig skin and doesn't know if she can stand to put one more into her mouth. Maybe she should run out to the market for some hot dogs or chicken wings. This way of losing weight isn't turning out to be as much fun as she thought it would.

Alice is well-versed on the weight-gaining consequences of eating fat. She can even rattle off exactly how many grams of the greasy stuff you'd consume in a handful of Hershey Reese's Pieces (10 grams), a tablespoon of regular salad dressing (7 grams), or a cheeseburger with fries (36 grams).

But despite her ever-expanding font of nutrition knowhow, Alice just hasn't managed to drop those 20 pounds that have been standing for years between her and a pair of size 10 jeans. So every now and then, she finds a brand-new fad diet bandwagon to jump on.

Which is how she came to be here, at her kitchen table at nine o'clock in the evening, facing down a bag of pork rinds. She never thought she'd be willing to kill for a nice, fresh tossed salad or a plain baked potato, but that's how she's feeling right now.

Like the Ghost of Fad Diets Past, the hunger gnawing at her stomach seems to bring back visions of all her previous frustrating attempts to lose weight: Her run for the Kaopectate after eating nothing but grapefruit for an entire day on a Hollywood-style diet. Choking down a glass of an energy-boosting, muscle-building liquid protein supplement on an empty stomach. And what *was* she thinking when she bought that mysterious fat-burning spray for $29.95, plus shipping, that promised to blast away unwanted pounds and inches an instant after she sprayed it into her mouth?

She figures she has lost and gained the same 10 to 20 pounds at least eight times. But she dreads the thought of remaining in the oversize-sweatsuit brigade.

So she's hanging her hopes on yet another diet—one more grab at that brass ring fantasy of a slinky, sylphlike new self. This time around, she's zapping the fat with a high-protein, low-carbohydrate regimen. If it worked for Aunt Helen, it can work for her.

Of course, there are trade-offs to consider. Just thinking about Aunt Helen's breath, which smells kind of like nail polish remover—a side effect of the diet—makes Alice queasy.

She leaps up from the table and throws open the pantry door. There it is: a box of linguine. She knows she shouldn't eat it, but she doesn't know if she can resist. She tears open the package.

The Problem with Fad Diets

According to a government survey, nearly 44 percent of us are trying to lose weight. The problem is how we're going about it. Of those who diet, only one-fifth are doing it the right way—by eating fewer calories and getting at least 2½ hours of activity a week. The rest of us, like Alice, are doing it the wrong way.

That comes as no surprise. We all know how monotonous it can be to monitor intake and measure portions.

The Hawaiian Diet: Back to Basics

The motto of the Hawaii State Department of Health's Nutrition Program: Traditional foods are best.

Too often, we turn to science for answers, especially when it comes to weight loss. We await the next big discovery for shedding pounds fast and easily. Native Hawaiians are taking a back-to-basics approach to combat a statewide obesity epidemic.

They're turning to the traditional foods that their ancestors thrived on—taro, sweet potatoes, breadfruit, bananas, and steamed fish—to lose weight and regain their health. The traditional Hawaiian diet is low in total fat (about 10 percent), high in complex carbohydrates (78 percent) and high in total fiber (30 grams per day) and contains an adequate amount of protein and minerals.

"This diet is what the Hawaiians practiced for centuries before Captain Cook's arrival," says Claire Hughes, R.D., Dr.P.H., chief of the health, promotion, and education branch of the Hawaii State Department of Health.

Obesity rates there have spiraled since the 1980s, as they have on the mainland. The problem, however, is worse among

And sometimes we get just plain worn-out from trying so hard. So it's easy to see why we're tempted by information that promises a quick fix.

Not only that, but many of us probably *will* lose weight on the average fabulous fad, for a very simple reason: We're eating fewer calories. No matter what regimen they prescribe, most fads simply restrict calorie intake in one way or another. So what's wrong with them, anyway?

native Hawaiians. About 50 percent are overweight or obese, compared with about 28 percent of the overall population. With the increasing obesity rate have come increasing rates of heart disease, diabetes, and other chronic illnesses.

"Captain Cook found healthy natives living here," explains Dr. Hughes. As the islands became more Westernized, in the mid-20th century, so did the diet of their people. Land development closed taro farms, fish ponds, and other food production areas that had been maintained by natives for centuries.

The traditional Hawaiian diet is a 3-week program conducted in groups of 25 to 30 people. Participants come to a community site for three meals a day prepared with traditional foods. One or two new vegetables are introduced each day. In all the programs, the overall health of the participants increased dramatically, in addition to their having lost weight.

While these community diet programs usually run for 3 weeks, Dr. Hughes stresses that the traditional Hawaiian diet is promoted as a lifelong program.

You can't stay on them. Because fad diets require drastic changes in your eating patterns, you just can't stay on them for long. "Fad diets usually last about a week. By week two, you're usually on the downside of the diet," says Melinda Manore, R.D., Ph.D., professor of nutrition at Arizona State University in Tempe.

Remember those pork rinds? Dr. Manore admits that she tried her share of fad diets before she became a nutritionist. In college, she went on a high-protein diet with her roommate. Since they didn't have a kitchen in their dorm room, the pair decided that their protein sources would be Vienna sausages and Kentucky Fried Chicken. For a week, they ate nothing except canned mini-wieners and cold fried chicken. And they lost weight. Her resolve vanished when she visited a friend who had just baked an apple pie. "I called my roommate and said, 'I don't care what you do, but I'm having a piece of pie.' And the diet was over," recalls Dr. Manore. She had lost 5 pounds, but by the next day, 3 of them had already come back.

You're more likely to gain it back. Fad diets don't teach good nutrition habits, which means that once the diet is over, most of the weight is regained, explains Dr. Manore. "The dieter learns nothing about good food choices or making long-term changes in diet and exercise habits." The result is that once you go off the diet, you slip back into your old habits—the same ones that caused you to gain weight in the first place.

You keep the fat and lose your muscle. When we talk about wanting to lose weight, what we really mean is that we want to lose fat. Well, that's not what you get on most fad diets, especially high-protein, no-carbohydrate plans, says Dr. Manore. The plunging needle on the scale isn't telling you what's going on *inside* your body.

Most of the weight lost on a no-carb diet is water. Here's why: Carbohydrates are our primary source of energy. And our bodies are able to store only a limited amount of this energy in the liver and muscle tissue—about 1,000 grams. For each gram of carbohydrate stored, we also store 4 grams of water. These water reserves are

The First Diet

Question: In 1880, if you refused an offer for a slice of apple pie because you were watching your weight, you would have said, "No thanks, I'm _____."

A. Dieting
B. Reducing
C. Banting
D. Torturing myself

The answer is C. The first modern-day diet was called banting, named for William Banting, a fashionable London undertaker who lost more than 50 pounds.

At age 65, Banting was so large that he could not tie his own shoes and had to walk down the stairs backward. Excess tissue in his throat pressed on his eustachian tubes and impaired his hearing. His doctor prescribed a diet nearly free of starch and sugar. Banting did so well on the diet of lean meat, dry toast, soft-boiled eggs, and green vegetables that by the following year he was down to a trim 150 pounds and could walk down the stairs forward. His hearing also returned.

Wanting to share his good news, Banting wrote up and printed 2,500 copies of his *Letter on Corpulence*. By the time he died, in 1878, more than 58,000 copies of his diet book had been sold, and *banting* had become the new lingo for reducing.

there to produce sweat, which helps us cool down when we exercise. When we restrict carbohydrate intake, our energy-starved bodies tap into those stored carbs. We find ourselves making more trips to the bathroom as our bodies get rid of all the water that was stored along with those carbs. And voilà! Weight loss.

We may feel pretty happy when we look at the scale and see a 6-pound loss after just a week of dieting. But less than a third of that weight is fat. You can double fat loss if you simply have a little patience and stick with a traditional low-calorie diet, says Dr. Manore.

They lack the essentials. Fad diets often eliminate entire food groups that provide essential nutrients, energy, and fiber. This isn't usually a problem since you can't stay on them long enough to develop a nutritional deficiency. Even so, it's a good idea to take a daily multivitamin supplement if you're dieting, says Dr. Manore. "Most dieters cannot meet the recommended vitamin and mineral requirements if they're consuming fewer than 1,200 to 1,600 calories a day," she says.

Most fads don't encourage physical activity. Fad diets almost never address the issue of exercise, yet it's an indispensable part of the healthy weight-loss equation. "After all these years, I'm convinced that exercise is the key to maintaining lean tissue when you're dieting. It's also the key to maintaining weight loss," says Dr. Manore. Ironically, when you're on a very low calorie fad diet, moving around is more difficult. Rigid diets often don't provide enough carbohydrate calories to fuel our brains or recharge our muscles. The result is that we feel like we need a dose of Geritol.

They can be bad for your health. Protein-rich diets tend to be chock-full of saturated fat and cholesterol, which can increase the risk of heart disease. When carb calories are drastically reduced, the body starts converting fatty acids into a fuel that the brain can use since not enough glucose is being provided by the diet. This process releases into the bloodstream chemicals called ketones, which can cause headaches, dizziness, fatigue, nausea, and bad breath. Too much protein can also tax the kidneys, which go into overdrive trying to process and excrete high levels of nitrogen and protein, explains Dr. Manore.

Sorting Fact from Fiction

Like lottery tickets and slot machines, fad diets appeal to our desire for an easy way out. We want to be thin, and we want it now. Which may explain why every year Americans plunk down $33 billion for weight-loss products and plans—often for gimmicks that simply don't work. Before you spend your hard-earned cash, learn to recognize some common weight-loss come-ons.

The diet claims that a particular miracle food burns fat. When it debuted, in the 1930s, the Hollywood Diet called for a few select vegetables, a small amount of protein, and lots of grapefruit, which was believed to contain a special fat-burning enzyme. The idea that grapefruit could speed up weight loss caught on and, over the years, spawned more than a dozen different diets starring the large, sometimes bitter citrus fruit.

Sure, grapefruit is fat-free, low in calories, and packed with vitamin C. Its high fiber and water content help fill you up. But does it stoke up your fat-burning furnace? Not a chance. "Foods don't burn fat. They create fat when we eat more calories than our bodies need," says Audrey Cross, Ph.D., nutrition professor at the Institute of Human Nutrition at Columbia University in New York City.

The all-you-can-eat diet. The soup du jour served at this all-you-can-eat buffet is stewed from a head of cabbage and flavored with onions, celery, green peppers, and a packet of onion soup. You can spoon up as much as you want for 7 days on the cabbage soup diet, which falsely claims that it was a healthy way for heart patients to lose up to 17 pounds prior to surgery.

She Gave Up on Fads and Lost Weight

According to her calculations, Barbara Cady, a former college instructor from Fairmont, West Virginia, who first joined TOPS in 1964, lost and gained about 900 pounds on fad diets over the course of 35 years.

Most things worked short-term, but never for the long term, Cady discovered. When she finally gave up on the quick-fix approach for good, she came up with a plan that she could live with for life, and she lost 47 pounds. Here's her advice.

Forget about prescribed diets, and stick with a balance of the foods you enjoy. The trick is simply to eat less of them. "Weight loss is a journey. And it's essential that you enjoy that journey if you're going to stick with it to the end," says Cady.

She found a way to enjoy her favorite—pizza—and still lose weight. Instead of ordering a thick crust, Barbara now orders thin crust. Then she tops it with loads of veggies, and maybe a little Canadian bacon, and skips the pepperoni and sausage.

"I understand now that weight control is not just about one thing. It's about all things," she says.

The bottom line is that any diet that calls for bizarre quantities of one type of food—whether it's cabbage soup, rice, or steak—violates the first basic principle of good nutrition: to balance your diet with a variety of foods, says Dr. Cross. Diets like these are so boring that you simply end up eating fewer calories.

Nutrients are cast as heroes and villains. Beware of fad diets that resemble a Saturday-morning cartoon, with one nutrient pitted against another. Instead of Superman, Batman, and Wonder Woman, the starring players are proteins, carbohydrates, fats, and (on rare occasions) alcohol—the four sources of calories in our diet. The scenario usually goes something like this: Nutrient A is the cause of all your weighty woes. Nutrient B is the solution to your troubles. A dietary version of the old blame game.

"We love to buy into this idea that there's something metabolically wrong with us that a certain combination of foods can fix," says Dr. Manore.

Since the mid-1980s, we've seen fat typecast as our nutritional arch villain. If you wanted to be thin, a low-fat diet was your ticket. You could eat what you wanted, as long as it didn't have fat. But it turned out that all the fat-free food we loaded up on was still chock-full of calories and only made us fatter.

In the backlash, carbohydrates became the new dietary villian, fueling a flurry of fresh fads with names like Sugar Busters!, Protein Power, the Carbohydrate Addict's Diet, and the Atkins Diet. All of these diets cast protein as the new nutritional superhero and fat as its friendly sidekick.

And so it goes. The cycle repeats itself over and over. Fat, protein, carbohydrate—who will be the bad guy next?

Rapid weight loss is the promise. *Lose 30 pounds in 30 days.* Maybe you've seen this claim or one similar to it and been tempted to try it out. This is a classic case of "if it sounds too good to be true, it probably isn't true," says Denise Bruner, M.D., president of the American Society of Bariatric Physicians and a physician practicing in Arlington, Virginia.

The truth is that it's physically impossible to lose 30 pounds of fat in 30 days. To lose weight, you have to create a calorie deficit, either by lowering your calorie intake or by burning up more calories through increased physical activity. You need a deficit of 3,500 calories to lose 1 pound. To lose 30 pounds, you would need a deficit of 105,000 calories. A person eating 2,800 calories a day takes in 84,000 calories in a month. The bottom line is that you could stop eating and still would have to burn an additional 21,000 calories to lose 30 pounds in 30 days. That's about 70 hours of brisk walking. You can see how ridiculous a claim like this is once you do the math.

Finding Out the Truth

The first problem with going *on* a diet is that sooner or later you'll have to go *off* that diet. Instead, you need to look for a lifelong approach to weight management, but how can you tell whether a program has live-with-it-for-life potential? Take this quick quiz from Ann Ruelle, R.D., of Advanced Healthcare, S.C., in Milwaukee and coauthor of the TOPS Club guide, *The Choice Is Yours.*

How does this affect my food choices? Fads tend to limit our food choices. Look for a plan where anything goes. You can't go through the rest of your life without eating your favorite foods. All foods should be legal.

Is this difficult to implement? Some diets call for hard-to-find foods or hard-to-follow regimens. For example, the Sugar Busters! plan suggests eating alligator, elk, and quail. Can you find these meats in your local grocery store?

Losing weight is difficult enough. The easier a program is to follow, the more likely you'll be to stick with it, says Ruelle.

Would this program affect my health? The next thing you should consider is the health benefits of a diet. Can you answer, "Yes, I will be better off than I am today because this plan will benefit my health"?

Would it control my weight? This is actually the last point to ponder, not the first, says Ruelle. Before you can start to think about weight loss in terms of numbers on a scale, you need to decide to change your lifestyle. And that lifestyle change needs to be one that is not just effective but also good for you in the long run.

Taking Personal Inventory

Who are you?

No, don't list your physical attributes, job, and number of kids. Who are you *really*? Until you can answer that question with the kind of soul-searching self-evaluation and honesty it requires, you'll never be permanently successful in your weight-loss quest.

"You really have to get acquainted with yourself," says Cheryl Rock, Ph.D., associate professor of family and preventive medicine at the University of California, San Diego. "This personal assessment is the absolute first and most important step in the weight-loss process."

You need to know where you are before you can decide where to go. You need to look at your eating patterns, think about the ways you like to have fun, and understand how you react to stress. You need to consider whether your goals are realistic and whether you're ready to take the time to achieve them.

So get a pencil and paper and spend some time with someone you may barely know—yourself.

How Much Weight Do You Need to Lose?

This is the first question you should ask when you tackle a weight-loss program, says Howard J. Rankin, Ph.D., behavioral psychology advisor for the TOPS Club and author of 7 Steps to Wellness. "The question should be 'What level of eating and exercise can I realistically expect to maintain?' The secret to being successful at weight control is to recognize what is possible for you and to set up your program accordingly."

For instance, if you're currently eating an average of 2,500 calories a day and the couch has a permanent imprint of your body, then deciding to suddenly go on a 1,200-calorie diet and jog 2 miles a day is probably a recipe for failure.

So start small and move up incrementally. Instead of declaring, "I'm going to eat healthier and exercise more," make a pact with yourself to eat at least ½ cup of vegetables each day. Or exercise an additional 5 minutes every other day. When you can count these small successes, it's easier to overlook the inevitable backsliding, says Sandra Haber, Ph.D., a New York City psychologist who specializes in women's weight issues.

And whether you're trying to drop 5 pounds or 50, don't overrate the importance of that goal, says Dr. Haber. "The idea of judging yourself by a number on the scale is a very important thing *not* to do," she says. "Weight is just one component of who you are, how you appear to others, and how you appear to yourself."

Focusing all your energy on reaching a goal weight and then not getting there—or not getting there fast enough—can feel overwhelming. The result is that you're more likely to give up, says Dr. Rankin. And this is going to take time. For instance, a moderately active woman who eats 1,200 calories a day will probably lose 3 pounds a month.

Are You Doing This for Yourself?

If you're trying to shed pounds because other people think you should or because a family member has been bugging you about it, you're less likely to succeed than if you're doing it for yourself.

Know Your BMI

Body mass index (BMI) is a more valuable measurement of health risks than your bathroom scale. Higher BMI numbers are associated with greater death rates and risk of diseases, including high cholesterol and blood pressure, heart disease, stroke, diabetes, and certain cancers.

Here's how to calculate your BMI.

1. Multiply your weight in pounds by 0.45 and then round it to the nearest whole number. For example, 150 pounds × 0.45 = 68. This number represents how much you weigh in kilograms.
2. Multiply your height in inches by 0.025. For example, if you're 5 feet 6 inches tall (66 inches), 66 × 0.025 = 1.65, your height in meters.
3. Square the answer from step 2: (1.65 × 1.65) = 2.72
4. Divide the answer in step 1 by the answer in step 3: (68 ÷ 2.72 = 25). This is your BMI.

A healthy BMI should fall below 25 advises Carol Boushey, Ph.D., assistant professor in the department of foods and nutrition at Purdue University in West Lafayette, Indiana. If you score 25 or more, you should lose enough weight to lower your BMI at least one or two numbers.

For clues about your motivation, listen to what you say. For example, when you told your best friend about your weight-loss plan, did you say, "I *should* lose weight" or "I *want* to lose weight"?

"When you hear someone say, 'I should lose weight,' that's usually a bad sign," says Dr. Haber. "*Should*s tend to be things that we think in our heads that we may or may not do. I *should* because it's healthy, or I *should* because I'll look better or because I can't zip my pants anymore. There's a lot of *should*s in life, and we don't do most of them."

Saying "want," however, signifies that you're doing this for yourself—and that's an important first step in losing weight.

Is This the Right Time to Make Changes?

Timing is everything when you're charting your weight-loss strategy. Are you in the middle of a kitchen remodeling job? Leaving in a couple of weeks for vacation? Then it's not the time to start changing your lifestyle habits.

"You want to embark on a weight-loss program when the rest of your life is as normal as possible," says Janet R. Laubgross, Ph.D., a clinical psychologist specializing in weight loss in Fairfax, Virginia.

Major changes in your life—like a new job, a move to a new residence, a marriage, or a divorce—raise your stress levels. If you pile more changes on top of that, such as a new exercise routine, you're likely to become overwhelmed and quit.

"Weight loss in itself is a stressor," says Dr. Laubgross. It gobbles up precious time in your already overbooked schedule. You may have to shop more frequently for fresh produce, carve 10 minutes from your lunch hour to take a walk, or sit down for a half-hour each week to plan healthy menus.

"When we ask ourselves if this is the right time, we should also be asking, 'Is this a time when I'm ready, willing, and able to take the time I need to make permanent lifestyle changes?'" says Dr. Laubgross.

Do You Know Your Favorites?

While it's important to eat low-calorie foods when you're trying to lose weight, it's much more important that you *like* those calories.

Too many women go on a diet, eating prescribed foods as if they were medicine—foods that they have no intention of eating after the diet is over. Then they can't wait to go off the program. So what's the point?

To design a program that includes foods you like best, rate the foods you eat on a scale of 1 to 10. A 1 is a food that you absolutely hate. A 10 is a food that you absolutely love. "I ask people to design diet programs with foods that are minimally a 6 and optimally a 10," says Dr. Haber. "We're looking for foods that nurture them, that taste good, and that they will continue to eat once they've lost the weight," she says. Now, if their top five foods are things like cheese puffs, chocolate cake, and Big Macs, Dr. Haber works with them to identify other, less fattening foods they also enjoy.

How Much Activity Do You Get?

Chances are, not enough. Only about one in four of us gets the 30 minutes of minimum daily activity that health experts recommend. Lack of activity is one of the main reasons we gain weight as we get older, says Miriam Nelson, Ph.D., associate chief of the Human Physiology Laboratory at the Jean Mayer USDA Human Nutrition Research Center on Aging at Tufts University in Boston and author of *Strong Women Stay Slim*.

Even if your job keeps you chained to your desk all day, you have to consciously choose ways to work activity back into your life, advises Dr. Nelson. You have to get up more, walk more, take the stairs more.

What's Your Body Image?

What do you see when you look in the mirror? In a survey conducted by *Psychology Today* magazine, 56 percent of women were dissatisfied with their appearance. Nearly two-thirds were dissatisfied with their weight.

But learning to like your body can double your chances of getting slimmer, say researchers at Stanford University School of Medicine. Here's how to get happy with your body *before* you lose weight.

Accept your power. Self-image has a lot to do with what you say to yourself internally, says Judy Schiller, Ph.D., a clinical social worker and psychoanalyst in San Francisco. Women who like their bodies tend to have an easier time losing weight. If a woman has a poor body image, the real problem is how she feels about herself. To be successful, she has to change the message to herself and say, "I am a good person, and I don't have to lose weight to feel valuable." Either way, she needs to take control of the situation and understand the underlying feelings that are getting in the way of controlling her weight. Then a weight control plan can be successful.

Get moving. To boost your body image and your confidence, get active. But community gyms aren't for everyone, says Michaela Kiernan, Ph.D., a behavioral scientist at Stanford University. You may be more likely to stick with a home-based fitness program, such as walking. That way, you don't have to face the stress or embarrassment of a group setting.

To get her clients moving, Dr. Haber asks them to pin-point the pleasure factor of various activities on a scale of 1 to 10. If you absolutely hate aerobics class, don't bother going. But if you love belly dancing, take a couple of classes. It's not important that aerobics burns more calories. What's important is finding an activity that will stay on your calendar and fit into your lifestyle.

How Supportive Is Your Environment?

"Think about the people in your environment," says Dr. Rankin. Make a list of who is supportive and positive and who is sabotaging you. One person could be both. Maybe you and your husband enjoy dinner out three or four nights a week. He may not want you to change your eating habits if it means that he has to change his routine, too. On the other hand, he may help you work in physical activity by asking you to go for a walk after dinner.

Decide how you're going to handle those situations. Overall, you really do need support if you're going to change your lifestyle. Women tend to do better at weight loss when they have some type of support network, so ask for it. Maybe you can get it from people at home, your friends, your coworkers, or a group like TOPS, says Dr. Rankin.

Do You Expect to Be a Perfect Dieter?

Let's say you have a party and a friend brings your favorite dessert—apple pie. You can't resist, and you have not one but two pieces. "I really blew it today," you say to yourself. You now have two choices: You can get rid of the leftover pie and go back on your program the next morning. Or you can figure "what's the use?" and eat the rest of the pie. Too many people do the latter. Weight-loss experts call it the I'll-diet-tomorrow effect.

The true problem isn't the extra piece of pie. "What really counts is how quickly you get back on your feet," says Dr. Haber.

So don't berate yourself. "Being a harsh, critical taskmaster never does anybody any good," she says. "It doesn't boost you up. It's defeating and negative."

Instead, find a way to deal with the situation in the most positive, optimistic way you can. In the apple pie situation, you can learn from the problem and offer to make the dessert next time.

Can You Remember Everything You Ate Today?

If the answer is no, you're not paying enough attention to what you're putting in your mouth. Unconscious eating is one of the primary reasons people gain weight, according to Audrey Cross, Ph.D., nutrition professor at the Institute of Human Nutrition at Columbia University in New York City.

We eat in front of the television or while we're standing at the kitchen sink. We wolf down fast food in the car. "The irony is that most people don't really enjoy what they are eating when they eat this way. That's why we eat so much," says Dr. Cross.

To eat less and enjoy it more, you need to find out how much you're eating on a regular basis. The best way to do this is to record everything you eat for the next few days. "When my clients do this, they're amazed at how much they eat," says Dr. Cross.

Do You Eat When Bored or Stressed?

Emotional overeating protects us from tension and worries, explains Dr. Haber. "As strange as it seems, overeating can be calming; it 'works,' at least in the short run," she says. "And that's why it's a difficult cycle to break."

It's often easier and less upsetting to be angry with ourselves than it is to be tense and angry at an important person in our lives. Often, we transfer our feelings into emotional overeating. The distraction of food, repetitive

Women's Food Obsession

Women are taught to think about food from a very early age. By age 8 or 9, young girls already understand the connection between food and their bodies, and they often begin dieting. So there's an early understanding of food, weight issues, and how they are interrelated.

Then there's the role food plays in our daily lives. We're the caretakers and nurturers, and food is one way for us to show our families that we're taking good care of them. It's an inescapable element of our daily lives. We plan the menus, stock the pantry, and do most of the cooking.

Even if we're ordering takeout food from a restaurant, we're in charge of what the family will eat. Because we're constantly involved with it and always thinking about it, somewhere along the way, it's going to come up in our conversations.

Some men, on the other hand, don't have a clue. They don't usually care what they're eating, how it got there, or what preparation went into it. When they run out of bologna, they expect it to just magically reappear in the refrigerator. Then when they gain a few pounds, they wonder, "How did I gain this weight?"

Expert consulted: Sandra Haber, Ph.D., psychologist, New York City

chewing and swallowing, and obsessive thoughts of food are psychologically safer than confronting our feelings head-on.

The first step in breaking the emotional eating cycle is to understand what feelings you're avoiding, allow yourself to be upset, and then choose an alternative behavior, says Dr. Haber.

Do You Put Everyone Else's Needs First?

Is your pantry stocked with chips and cookies so the kids have something quick to snack on? Do you serve macaroni and cheese for dinner because it's the only thing everyone will eat without complaint? As women, we tend to put the needs and wants of others before ourselves. Our weight-loss efforts are easily defeated when we don't factor our own needs into the equation.

"It's a concept I call healthy selfishness," says Dr. Haber. "For most people in our culture, the word *selfish* has a very negative spin. And yet healthy selfishness is a key concept in self-esteem, in feeling good about yourself, and in making good things happen for yourself."

For example, if everyone in the family absolutely loves ice cream, we keep the fridge stocked with fudge ripple. If we don't eat the ice cream, we feel deprived. If we do eat it, we blow our daily calorie count. A better approach might be to buy a lower-calorie treat, like frozen yogurt, that everyone will enjoy just as much and that we can also eat.

PART TWO

The Major Keys
of Success

See Yourself Thin

The mind can lead the body to do amazing things. After downhill champion Picabo Street injured her knee in a 70 mph crash on the Colorado ski slopes in 1996, she had to make some serious changes in her training plans for the 1998 Olympics. She couldn't ski the course in a pre-Olympic race along with her competitors, so instead she watched videotapes, and she created an interactive CD-ROM skiing game wherein she coached her players. In her mind, she visualized skiing the Olympic course again and again.

Her mind led her body. Her reward: a gold medal in the 1998 Olympics in Nagano, Japan.

"When we create an image, it helps us focus. It puts our attention on turning the image into reality," explains Lynnette Young Overby, Ph.D., assistant professor of theater at Michigan State University in East Lansing, who has studied visualization and used it with her dance students.

If ballet dancers can master complicated routines and Olympic skiers can win the gold, all through the power of visualization, you can certainly use the same techniques to create a happier, more active, and thinner you.

The Mind–Body Partnership

You may think imagery exists only in your head, but your body knows better. When an athlete imagines sprinting to the finish line, the muscle fibers in her legs start twitching as if she were running an actual race.

The same principle applies to psychological goals, including weight loss. "You're preparing your subconscious mind through the medium of your conscious mind," says Jane Lincoln, who uses guided imagery at the George Washington University Center for Integrative Medicine in Washington, D.C. Once you've prepared yourself with an image of what you want to accomplish—whether that's finishing your first 5-K race or slipping into your sleekest black

Thin Is In—But Just for Women

For men, bulk is the buzzword. And if men can't have muscles, they'll take being a little bigger any way they can get it. For them, being big is about intimidation and strength.

Women, on the other hand, get the message that if you're thin, everything will be okay. Many of their ideals are built around thinness. A woman thinks, "If I were thin, I'd have a better job, I'd have a better love relationship, and I'd feel better about myself." True, those things may well happen when a woman loses weight because she pays more attention to her appearance. She holds her head higher, and she goes out of her way to meet people. She may attribute her new social success to weight loss, but her change in attitude may have played just as big a part.

Expert consulted: Tracy Sbrocco, Ph.D., assistant psychology professor, Uniformed Services University, Bethesda, Maryland

dress for the annual Christmas party—your body and mind can respond in ways that may turn your hopes into reality.

If you have a good imagination, you'll have no trouble using imagery to help you accomplish your weight-loss goals. But if you've never been able to picture yourself on the beach, feeling the sun on your face and hearing the sound of the waves rolling onto the sand, you might need to get your imagination into shape.

"Some people naturally form pictures in their minds. Some don't. But imagery is a skill that can be learned," says Kate Hays, Ph.D., a psychologist at the Performing Edge in Toronto, a company that coaches athletes, artists, and business people on improving their performance.

Fortunately, these "exercises" are fun. To test your visualization ability, try this: Think of a lemon. What does it feel like in your hand? What does the skin look like? Now slice the lemon in half. How does the fruity pulp smell? How does it taste?

After you've finished, think about which sensations seemed most vivid—or vaguest. This will give you some idea of which kinds of sensations will come naturally to you in your visualizations and which might need some sharpening up, Dr. Hays explains. Maybe you could see the lemon but not feel its pitted skin in your palm. Or maybe you could taste its sour juice but couldn't smell its fresh citrus scent. Learning your sensory strengths and weaknesses is important because of their impact on imagery—and your weight-loss success. The more senses you use in your visualizations, the more effective they'll be in helping you reach your goals.

Practice, Practice, Practice

"People say practice makes perfect," says Karen D. Cogan, Ph.D., assistant professor of psychology at the University of North Texas Center for Sports Psychology and Performance Excellence in Denton and a former competitive gymnast. "I say, 'Practice makes permanent.'" The more you use imagery, the more effective a part of your weight-loss toolbox it will become.

Here are some tips to get you started.

Be sense-ible. When you do imagery, draw on the traditional five senses: touch, taste, smell, sight, and sound. Then add one more: kinesthetic, or how your body feels when it moves.

Lincoln remembers one patient who, in her efforts to lose weight, drew upon her memories of being a dance major in college. "She visualized feeling graceful and strong. She pictured the room she used to dance in, right down to the smell of the wood floors. And she told herself, 'I was once that way; I can be that way again.'"

The more senses you involve in your visualizations—whether you're picturing yourself easily refusing second helpings of potato salad at the company barbecue or enjoying the extra energy that comes with a healthier lifestyle—the more powerful and effective your images will be in making your dreams come true.

Change perspectives. Sport psychologists talk about external imagery (where you see yourself performing an action as though you were watching yourself on TV) and internal imagery (where you imagine the experience through your own eyes). The more perspectives you can experience, the more powerful your imagery will be in motivating and supporting your progress toward the life you've always wanted to have.

Loosen up and breathe. Whatever senses or perspectives you choose to use in your imagery, make sure you're calm and relaxed before you begin.

To relax quickly and easily, try this breathing exercise, recommended by Simone Ravicz, Ph.D., a licensed clinical psychologist in Pacific Palisades, California, and author of *High on Stress*. Inhale for 5 seconds through your nose. Hold your breath for 20 seconds. Then exhale for 10 seconds through your nose, imagining all the stress melting away. It is important that you breathe from your

The Glories of Chocolate

Women have always known that chocolate soothes the heart. Scientists are finally catching on. Researchers have found that chocolate contains various health-promoting antioxidants as well as iron, chromium, copper, and magnesium.

Nibbling on chocolate doesn't have to torpedo your weight-loss plans. Here's how the sweet treat can deliver its magic without too many consequences.

Go gourmet. "If you must have chocolate, go for the very best chocolate available, in the smallest possible amount," says Laurel J. Branen, R.D., Ph.D., associate professor of food and nutrition at the University of Idaho in Moscow. (She admits to a weakness for the tiny Dove Promises.) Stay away from cheap chocolate and treat yourself to a truffle at the Godiva counter instead. You'll feel more satisfied and consume fewer calories.

Eat an ounce and stop. It takes about an ounce of chocolate to satisfy a craving and about 30 minutes for your body to realize it, Dr. Branen says.

Go fat-free. In blind taste tests at the University of Missouri in Columbia, people liked the taste of fat-free chocolate ice cream just as much as regular ice cream. Chocolate's complex flavor comes from a host of compounds, which makes it less vulnerable to "off" tastes in fat-free or low-fat foods.

diaphragm when you inhale so that your stomach rises, not your chest.

Imagining Your Life

Imagery can help you picture your ideal life and set weight-loss goals, but it can also work well for life's everyday challenges, from your workouts to your career. And it can help you cope when you're faced with a stressful situation that usually drives you to the cookie jar for relief. Just as a marathoner thinks through a race and all its possibilities, from rain to exhaustion and everything in between, you can prepare yourself mentally for dinner with Mom or a difficult meeting with your boss. The result? You'll respond differently and break the cycles that lead to emotion-induced eating.

A "Dream Album" Helped Her Lose

Sonia Turner, of Timmins, Ontario, had no trouble imagining herself in a bikini each time she went on a new diet. But the images of a thinner self never seemed to stick, and neither did her diet—until she started her "dream album." It gave her visual reminders of what she wanted to accomplish.

Sonia began her dream album with a photograph from her husband's company newsletter. "It was another Christmas when I didn't attend the company dance because I was too self-conscious about my weight," she says. Then the newsletter arrived, featuring photos of couples dressed to the nines as they dined and danced the night away at the holiday bash. Sonia decided she didn't want to miss out on the fun any longer. She cut out the pictures and pasted them in her album, adding a forecast for the

But it's not just about losing weight, says Dr. Ravicz. "It's about changing your lifestyle. We can create our own reality of what we want our lives to be like."

Perhaps you'd like to dust off your dancing shoes, plant a vegetable garden, or walk after dinner each night. "But I can't," you think. "I haven't danced in years, I know I won't have time to weed, and who will do the dishes?"

Well, just stop. Too often, negative thinking throws cold water on our ideas before we even have a chance to dream.

To get beyond those automatic thoughts, Dr. Ravicz recommends a visualization that she calls Playing Center Stage. Think of the person you would like to be. (Feel free to draw on the traits of people you admire, whether they're friends, family, public figures, or even fictional characters.)

following year: "And also in attendance were Doug and Sonia Turner."

She filled page after page with similar images of inspiration and motivation. She cut out a photo of a woman wearing jeans, something she hadn't been able to do since she was a teenager. She included magazine stories about women who had lost weight.

She applied the same philosophy toward exercise, pasting in her dream album photographs of speed walkers and runners. Now the woman who could barely walk around her block runs 5 miles daily and is training for a marathon.

One year and 115 pounds after making her resolution, Sonia went with her husband to his company's holiday dance.

What qualities would she have? How would she spend her time? How would she interact with other people? What would her job be? How would she dress? What habits would she have? How would she approach food?

Once you've fully envisioned your ideal self (using all your senses, of course), try actually living a week of your life in her shoes, acting just as you would expect her to act. Freed from the psychological constraints that we all put on our own behavior, you'll try new activities, meet new people, eat new foods, and experience (at least snippets of) a life that you'd only imagined.

Back to the Future

Now that you've whetted your creative appetite, it's time to harness the power of your imagination to create the most detailed, vivid picture of the healthier, active life that you plan to lead.

To create such a picture, pick a day in the future, perhaps a year from today. See yourself waking up, then let your imagination run wild, using the questions below as a starting point. You can, of course, replace these questions with your own to create a more personalized visualization script. Whatever you choose, you may want to record this into a tape recorder, leaving pauses after each question to allow yourself to think about your answers, suggests Dr. Hays.

Morning: How do you start your day? Do you roll out of bed an hour earlier so that you can exercise in the mornings? Do you stretch before you shower? How does it feel to move in your new, leaner body? What does the shower water feel like as it moves over your newfound physique? What outfit do you choose to wear? How does it fit? How does it feel against your skin? What emotions do you feel as you look in the mirror and see the result of your work?

What's the expression on your face? What does that high-fiber breakfast taste like?

Midmorning: How is your day going? What projects are you working on? What did you bring from home for your midmorning snack? How are you handling the stress of a busy morning? How are people reacting to your directions and ideas?

Noon: How will you use your lunch hour today? What food will you eat? How does it taste to you? How have you made your lunch hour more active? Will you go for a walk after a healthy lunch or perhaps even jog a few miles with a like-minded colleague? What do the outdoors sound like after the hum of your computer? How does it feel to leave work and be active? How does it feel to return to your desk after spending 20 minutes burning calories and stress?

Midafternoon: How are you dealing with the midafternoon slump? How are you managing the day's workload? How are you handling people's demands?

Early evening: How do you feel after a day's work? Do you go directly home, or do you stop at the gym for a quick spin on the stationary bike? What do you do after you arrive home? How do you handle the postwork (and postworkout) munchies? What are your plans for dinner? Will you be dining with your family or hosting friends? What are you (or your spouse) cooking? What aromas can you smell? When you sit down for your meal, what room in your house are you sitting in? What does the table look like? How is the food on your plate arranged? When you take your first bite, how does it taste? What do you talk about at dinner? What (if anything) do you serve for dessert? What are your after-dinner plans?

Night: When you get ready for bed, what pajamas do you choose? As you crawl into bed, how do you feel? What are you thinking as your head hits the pillow and your eyes close?

After you finish this visualization, consider the images that came to mind. Then grab a pen and paper and start thinking of how you can make this mental picture come true. Hays suggests jotting down the baby steps that you can immediately take toward your goal.

Maybe you want to run a 5-K with your daughter, but the most exercise you get right now is carrying laundry between the bedrooms and the basement. What's the midpoint between yourself right now and the ideal life you pictured just a few minutes ago? After mulling it over, you decide that walking a 5-K represents the midpoint. What can you do to reach that spot between today and the future?

Perhaps you can start by walking for 5 minutes when you have some free time during your day, then adding minutes and miles until you reach 3.2 miles (the length of a 5-K). How can you go from that midpoint to your ideal? Maybe you decide to mix walking and running, and devise a training program that gradually brings you to the race date. Through the strength of your own mental images, you can propel your mind and body toward a healthier, slimmer you.

Dressing Up to Slim Down

Marilyn Monroe was undoubtedly one of the most beautiful women of the 20th century. She was a cinema goddess and a sex symbol. She was also a size 16.

"Women who look good all the time aren't necessarily thin or gorgeous," says Gale Grigg Hazen, a color and image consultant in Saratoga, California, and author of *Fantastic Fit for Every Body.* "But they spend time on themselves, and they pay attention to what looks good on them."

That's hard for most of us. We often feel guilty spending time or money on ourselves, and we may not even know what works best on our fuller figures. We tell ourselves that we'll just wait until we lose weight, and then we'll buy new clothes.

Wrong approach.

Dressing well is just as important as eating healthy. "It's another way of nourishing yourself," says Ruth P. Rubinstein, professor of sociology at the Fashion Institute of Technology in New York City and author of *Dress Codes.* What's more, the better you look and feel about yourself, says Hazen, the more successful you'll be at losing weight. "If you dress well, you look good immediately. It's not something you have to wait 6 months to lose weight for," says DeeDee, a top plus-size model with the Ford modeling agency in New York City.

So start wearing clothes that flatter your figure now, *before* you shed a single pound.

Clean Out Your Closet

Before you rush out and buy a new wardrobe, check what's hiding in your closet. Chances are you have some real treasures in there, as well as some that you'd swear were snuck in by aliens.

Here's how to weed out the good from the bad and the downright ugly.

Invite a friend. Closet cleaning should be fun, says Francine Taylor, stylist of ABC's morning show *The View*. The two of you could put on some dance music and pretend you're shopping at a fancy boutique. Tell a story about each garment—where you bought it, who you kissed while you were wearing it, what special thing happened to you in it. And don't forget your dresser drawers.

Divide it up. Toss everything into one of three piles— looks great; needs repair; trash—so that everything you put back will look fabulous, Hazen says.

Donate it. Those bell-bottoms? That orange rayon dress? The peasant blouse? They're history. Drop them off at a local charity. You'll free up space in your closet and make it easier to find the clothes you do wear, Taylor says. Plus, there's the tax deduction.

If the shoe *doesn't* fit, chuck it. Resist holding on to things from your thinner days. The goal is to have a closet full of clothes that fit and flatter your body *right now*, not to have constant reminders that you're not the weight you want to be. When you get to that weight, you'll have an excuse to go shopping.

Take the 1-year test. Get rid of anything that leaves you thinking, "But it looked good on the mannequin." Don't kid yourself. If you haven't worn it in a year, you're probably never going to wear it again, says Hazen.

What Men Think

The old saying "You can't be too thin" doesn't hold true with many men. They still prefer their women larger than we think they do. The proof: When men choose from a range of body shapes that they think are attractive, they pick larger silhouettes than women think men prefer.

So why don't women feel like goddesses when they have curves that would make Rita Hayworth swoon? Because that's not today's fashion. The ideal body type seen on television and in magazines is such an unrealistically thin standard that even models and actresses must work unbelievably hard to live up to it.

Because most of us are shorter and heavier than a 5-foot-9-inch supermodel with "perfect" 34-24-34 measurements, we end up feeling bad about our bodies, regardless of how many times our husbands compliment our shapes. If we recognize that we tend to have distorted images of ourselves and stop trying to meet the unrealistic expectations we think others have of us, we can more easily work toward self-acceptance.

Expert consulted: Stacey Tantleff Dunn, Ph.D., assistant professor of psychology, University of Central Florida and director of the Laboratory for the Study of Eating, Appearance, and Health, Orlando

Stash it away. If you can't bear to part with certain things, pack them in a box, then date it and store it. If you haven't missed anything in the box after 6 months, haul it off to Goodwill.

Take it to a tailor. Put aside anything that's missing a button or needs to be altered. If you can't make the repairs yourself, find a good seamstress.

Organize it. At this point, all that's left are outfits that make you look great. So hang like items together—all your pants, shirts, dresses, skirts—arranging them from darkest to lightest colors. "When your clothes are organized, it's easy to see what pieces are missing," Taylor says. Perhaps you don't have a black jacket, or you look great in yellow but don't have a single top in that color. Learning what's in your closet helps you decide what items you need and saves you from buying red shirt number three.

Make a list. Attach pen and paper to the back of your closet door and jot down missing items as they occur to you. It's much easier to remember that you need a brown belt when you're getting dressed and realize that all you have is black.

Mark your calendar. Now that your closet is neat and tidy, the key to keeping it that way is to check back every 3 months. It's like cleaning out your refrigerator (only there shouldn't be anything moldy to throw out). Note any new items you need, and check the condition of the things you wear frequently. Collar fraying on your favorite white blouse? Toss it and get a new one.

Now it's time to fill in the holes.

Take the Misery out of Shopping

Most women love to shop. The problem is that when you're overweight, the thought of trying on clothes under harsh fluorescent lighting in front of cheap, three-way mirrors in overheated dressing rooms is enough to send you screaming for chocolate. Well, there's a way to deal with that problem. If you try on only the clothes that are right for you, you may be surprised at what your reflection shows. "By using a few fashion tricks, you can look up to 20 pounds thinner," says Diane Irons, an international image consultant to celebrities and models and author of *911 Beauty Secrets*. Here are some of the tricks she's talking about.

Bring your best friend. Husbands won't do. They have too much at stake to be totally honest. You need someone who's not afraid to tell you that those pants aren't the most flattering on you or that sleeveless shirts don't make the most of your shape. Otherwise, you'll wind up with another outfit you'll never wear.

Get comfortable. Wear an outfit that's easy to take off, such as a button-up blouse, slip-on shoes, and pull-on pants. And wear the right things *under* your clothes, including panty hose and a well-fitted bra. "They'll have a tremendous effect on the way the clothes fit," Hazen says.

Resist buying on impulse. When you buy something on a whim, there's a good chance that it won't match anything in your closet once you get it home. Make a shopping list before you leave the house so that you have a clear idea of what you're looking for.

Take a tote. Bring with you anything you're trying to match. That way, you're not guessing at colors, and you can make sure the item you're buying works with what you already have. Also, bring shoes to try on with the outfit and a comb or brush to fix your hair between outfits.

Test the fit. Wearing clothes that fit well is the single most important step to looking good, says Hara Estroff Marano, author of *Style Is Not a Size*. "Clothes that are too tight or too big make you look larger than you really are."

- Shirts or blouses: Reach both arms above your head to see if you have enough room under the arms. Also, make sure that there's no tugging around your bust and that when you put your arms down, the sleeves fall around your wrist bone.
- Jackets and overblouses: They should end at your hips. Most important, the shoulder line should be just at the edge of your shoulders. "Shoulders really have to fit neatly. They can't be sloppy, because the shoulder line creates the dominant line in a garment," Marano says.
- Pants, skirts, and dresses: Bend down as if you're picking something up off the floor. If there's a chair or bench in the dressing room, sit down. You should have enough room to move around freely without feeling as if something might pop or tear, says Irons.
- Waists: To check the fit, slip two fingers in the waistband. Pull ½ inch of fabric out at both hips to make sure that it's not too tight. And before buying the dress or pants, check to make sure that the back looks as good as the front.

Size things up. Be open to trying on several sizes. Are size 16 pants too long? Try a 16 petite. Is size 12 a bit snug? Try a 14. Don't get upset if you have to go up a size, Hazen says. Your size is bound to be different from one clothing line to the next because there's no set standard for sizing among manufacturers. Besides, the size on the tag isn't what matters. "Don't go for the size; go for the fit," she advises.

Ask for help. The salesclerk can be your best ally. If the store doesn't have something in your size, the clerk may know when they'll be getting more, or she can call around to other stores to find it, DeeDee says. They'll call you when it comes in.

Lower your expectations. Clothes are cut for the "average" woman. The problem is that there is no average woman. That's why it's so hard to find clothes off the rack that fit perfectly. "If you expect that most things won't fit, you won't get frustrated and quit," Hazen says. Instead, you'll be delighted when you find one or two things that do fit well.

Styles to Suit Your Shape

The secret to looking spectacular no matter what your size or shape is to show off your best features, DeeDee says. If you have great legs, wear skirts hemmed above the knee. Gorgeous eyes? Wear, close to your face, something that matches their color.

"You don't have to be cookie-cutter pretty to look pretty amazing," Irons says.

If you're not sure what your best features are, ask someone you love and trust. Then use these fashion-forward tips and garment-by-garment guide to find a look that you can love.

Create a signature style. Once you find a look that works for you, duplicate it. "I call it developing a uniform," Hazen says. A uniform makes picking out something to wear a snap. DeeDee, for example, always wears black pants and dress boots with a V-neck cashmere sweater or a blouse with a shell underneath.

Start with seven. To build a beautiful wardrobe, start with these basic pieces: a white shirt; a gray pants suit; a sweater; a black skirt, jacket, and pants; and black boots or heels. "You can make it through a whole year just by mixing these seven pieces," Taylor says. The sweater should be a color that looks good on you, she adds, and it can be a cardigan, V-neck, or turtleneck—whatever flatters you most.

To add variety to your wardrobe, accessorize with scarves, jewelry, and different types of tops. But stick to items that are classic, rather than trendy. "The trendy items will be out of style in a few months, but classics never go out of style," Taylor says.

Find the right fabric. Stay away from those that cling rather than drape, stiff materials that form harsh lines or boxy looks, and bulky clothes that add visual pounds, Marano says. Stick with fabrics that create smooth, clean lines, like wool and silk crepes, Lycra, cotton and rayon blends, and gabardine. They may cost a little more, but they're a better investment in the long run.

Pick small prints. Somewhere, we got the idea that we should never wear prints. "You *can* wear prints—just choose smaller patterns and make sure that the print is on the slimmest part of your body," Irons says. So if you're wider at your hips than your chest, wear a printed top with a solid skirt.

Fix the fit. Sleeves that are too long can easily be shortened, and roomy pants can be hemmed or taken in. These alterations make a world of difference, Hazen says. You instantly go from looking sloppy to looking put together.

Stick with steam. Wrinkles ruin the drape of a garment. To keep clothes wrinkle-free, hang them up as soon as you take them off. Still wrinkled? Use a hand steamer instead of an iron. It's quicker, and the moisture prevents static cling, says Julie Alderfer, head of wardrobe for the television program *The View*. Or hang your clothes in the bathroom when you shower, and let the steam do its work.

Blouses and Tops

Whether you're full-busted or flat as Kansas, what you wear on top can serve to enhance your look. Here's how.

Know your necklines. V-neck and surplice necklines are especially slimming, Marano says, because they create vertical and diagonal lines that make you look longer and thinner through the torso.

Slim with sleeves. Tapered sleeves make your arms look longer and more slender, Marano says. Sleeves with broad cuffs, however, shorten the line of the arm and add weight to your hips when your arms are at your sides.

Reshape your shoulders. Give rounded shoulders a more flattering shape by choosing set-in sleeves rather than drop sleeves, Marano says. Set-in sleeves attach at the shoulder, whereas drop sleeves start below the shoulder. Shoulder pads can also reshape shoulders and make your upper body look more proportionate with your hips. But bigger is not better. "They only add bulk," says Irons. Replace large pads with small round ones that conform to your shoulders, she suggests. Look for them at sewing and fabric stores.

Pass on pockets. If you're full-figured, avoid wearing shirts or blouses with breast pockets. They'll only make you look bigger, Irons says. By the same token, you can maximize a small bosom with breast pockets and large shirt buttons.

To tuck or not to tuck. If you have a defined waist, tucking in your shirt creates a flattering hourglass shape, DeeDee says. But avoid this trick if you're larger around the middle.

Grow with a tank. If you're short-waisted, wearing a silk, satin, or knit tank top under a jacket adds length to your neck and torso, Taylor says.

Jackets

A good-quality jacket is a key staple in every woman's wardrobe. "It takes you everywhere," Irons says. You can wear it with a skirt or pants, or even over a dress. And unlike other articles of clothing, jackets can be tailored many times, which is handy when you're losing weight. Here are Irons's suggestions for finding the right jacket for your wardrobe.

Pick the perfect cut. If you're large-busted, avoid double-breasted jackets and breast pockets. They make full-figured women appear larger than they are. Instead, go with a tuxedo-cut jacket, which will make you look taller and thinner.

Seek out seams. Look for a jacket that has a line of buttons or vertical seams down the front. These elements visually lengthen your torso and have a slimming effect.

Trim with a nip and a tuck. Jackets with a gently nipped-in waist trim the middle of your body and are very stylish.

Vanity Sizing?

We all know the exhilaration of slipping into a pair of jeans that are a size smaller than normal. That number on the tag says we're thinner than we thought. If only it were true.

The sobering news is that our clothes are growing with us. A size-12 woman in the 1950s had a 24-inch waist. Today it's 28.

As our bodies grew over the decades, so did our sensitivity about the number on the size tag. So clothing manufacturers learned that a size-12 woman would be more likely to buy jeans if she could fit into a size 10, says Margaret Voelker-Ferrier, chairperson of the fashion design program at the University of Cincinnati.

We've become so obsessed with size that many of us

Consider a knit. A knit jacket won't wrinkle and can be very slimming if it skims the body rather than clings to it.

Dresses and Skirts

There's much to consider when choosing skirts and dresses. What are your hips like? Your stomach? Your waist? Your answers will determine what you buy.

Forgo flared. A-line and flared silhouettes add width to your hips. Instead, choose skirts and dresses that are tapered slightly in from the hips. "A tapered skirt really flatters your legs and gives your body a very long, narrow look," Marano says.

Show some leg. If you have great legs, draw attention to them by wearing skirts and dresses hemmed above the

refuse to buy anything bigger than the magic number we've set for ourselves, she says.

We're paying a price for that smaller number. A roomier size 8 costs more than a "true" size 8, says Gale Grigg Hazen, a color and image consultant in Saratoga, California, and author of *Fantastic Fit for Every Body.*

But don't be surprised if you order your wedding dress two sizes larger than you think you wear. Wedding dresses are still cut to the standards of the 1950s, when a 12 was today's size 8, says Hazen.

To avoid letting vanity sizing affect you, stop worrying about what the tag says. "Concentrate on what fits and flatters you, even if that means your blouse, skirt, and jacket are all different sizes," Hazen says.

knee. If you're short, stick with longer skirts to make you look taller and thinner.

Slim with a slit. A front slit creates a long vertical line that is very slimming, Irons says.

Wrap it up. Wrap skirts are another slimming choice because they form a long vertical line where the two skirt panels overlap, Marano says.

Pants

Ever put on a pair of pants that fit yet didn't do you justice? Whether you're looking for jeans or dress pants, these tips will help you pick a pair that flatters your figure.

Play it straight. Bell-bottoms may have made their way back into style, but you don't have to be an enabler of bad fashion. Stick with straight-leg pants, Irons says, for a slimming line.

Get hip. If you're trying to minimize your hips, pick pants without hip pockets, Taylor says.

Pass on pleats. Pleats draw attention to your tummy. Enough said.

Know whether to buckle up. If you have a defined waist, wearing a belt will accentuate the positive, Taylor says, but belts are usually unflattering for women with larger waists.

Show Your True Colors

Color is the pizzazz that makes an ordinary outfit extraordinary. And while some colors are slimming, others add pounds. Here's how to use the colors in your wardrobe to enhance your figure.

Top it off. Wear bright colors on top and dark colors on the bottom to bring people's attention upward. "If you wear a turquoise shirt with black pants, for example, their eyes will be drawn to your face," Taylor says.

Wear just one. Wearing the same color from your shoulders to your shoes—called monochromatic dressing—streamlines your body by creating one long vertical line.

Match it up. Match your panty hose to your shoes. It provides that same slimming line of color, Irons says.

Begin with basics. Start with neutral classics in black, gray, navy, brown, and khaki, then accessorize with color. To add a splash of color, wear a bright top under a jacket, tie a colorful scarf around your neck, or pick an eye-catching purse. "I wear a lot of black, so I get pocketbooks in wacky colors," Marano adds. "It's a modern look and an inexpensive way to update your wardrobe."

Add the Finishing Touches

It's the last thing we do before we run out the door: Throw on some earrings, maybe even a necklace, and grab our purse. But these shouldn't be last-minute decisions. "Looking your best is all in the details," Hazen says. Here's how to accessorize your slimming wardrobe with style.

Scarf it up. Knot a long scarf at midchest to trim and elongate your torso. "Go for colorful scarves, because next to your face is a great place to put color," Marano says.

Slenderize with buttons. A vertical line of buttons down the front of a blouse, jacket, or dress is very slimming. "Try replacing the standard buttons with gold or silver ones to really enhance the look of a solid-color suit," Marano says.

Forget about flats. Flat shoes really do nothing for you, Irons says. Heels, however, provide an elegant look that lengthens your legs. For added stability, stick with a chunky heel rather than a stiletto.

Size it right. Larger women can carry off larger accessories, like chunky earrings or bracelets. But use some restraint. "You want your jewelry to be noticeable, but that doesn't mean it should be monstrously large," Marano says.

Go long. When wearing a necklace, choose a pendant on a long chain to lengthen and slim your torso, Irons says.

Keep it simple. Whether it's a pin on your lapel or a bangle bracelet, it's better to wear one piece of striking jewelry than several smaller pieces. "A simple, unencumbered look is very modern," Marano says.

Pick a petite purse. Full-figured women should stick with handbags that are no larger than 10 by 13 inches, Irons says. Anything bigger just adds girth.

Wear the right undergarments. Your bra is one of the most important things you put on. Its fit determines the drape of your sweater or blouse. If you're like most women, you're still trying to squeeze into that 34B you wore when you were 20. In fact, 8 out of 10 women are wearing the wrong-size bra, Irons says.

If you haven't been professionally fitted in the past 3 years or so, it's time to get rechecked. You can get fitted free of charge at most department stores.

Emotional Eating

For Jan McBarron, M.D., brown sugar was the last straw. As she stood in her kitchen one midnight, scooping the sweet stuff out of the box with a tablespoon, she thought: "I can't *believe* I'm doing this." Miserable and 70 pounds overweight, the premed student put down the spoon.

"I was very unhappy, and my weight reflected it," says Dr. McBarron, now director of Georgia Bariatrics, a medical center for overweight people in Columbus, Georgia, and cohost of the nationally syndicated health talk show *Duke and the Doctor*. A nurse at the time, she was so dissatisfied with her career that she turned to food for solace.

Yet as her weight rose, her self-esteem plummeted, sending her into a spiral of increasing job frustration, followed by more overeating, followed by more weight gain.

"Like most overweight people, I was trying to feed emotions," she says. Now 70 pounds lighter, Dr. McBarron speaks from experience when she tells her patients that the excess weight often isn't the problem; the hidden emotions are.

Eating instead of Feeling

For some, it's alcohol or drugs; others escape into work or exercise to avoid feelings that they can't handle. For many overweight women, the "drug" of choice is food.

"People who use food to numb out are usually eating to manage negative feelings," says Marlene Schwartz, Ph.D., codirector of the Center for Eating and Weight Disorders at Yale University.

You may feel lonely, angry, or frustrated. Perhaps you're undergoing a major life change—children leaving home, divorce, a career switch. "That's when women are likely to overeat as a way of comforting themselves," says Dr. Schwartz.

This isn't necessarily bad. "To some degree, we all use food for comfort, both physically and psychologically," says Ronni M. Kahn, Ph.D., a psychologist with the Eating Disorders Program of the Richard Young Center in Omaha, Nebraska. Think back on the cup of hot chocolate that comforted you on a cold winter's day or the pint of Häagen-Dazs that got you through the breakup with your college boyfriend.

"That's okay," says Dr. Kahn, "unless you reach the point where every hurt, every anger, every everything, calls for food. When eating is the only way you can cope, that's a danger signal."

This behavior is frequently found in women with binge-eating disorder, characterized by eating enormous amounts of food within a very short time period. A classic binge might include an entire pizza, a liter of soda, and a gallon of ice cream within an hour.

Asked how they feel after binges, women often answer, "I don't know. I didn't feel anything. I didn't even taste the food," says Dr. Schwartz. "It's as though the extreme overeating is used to escape the awareness of whatever feelings they were having."

"Most women who overeat don't even see the connection between what they're feeling and their running to the refrigerator," says Cynthia G. Last, Ph.D., author of *The Five Reasons Why We Overeat*.

Why Can't We Live on Love Alone?

Popular songs, movies, and literature glorify the idea of love as an appetite suppressant. Could it be the answer to weight loss?

Maybe. For a little while.

For women who have been focused on weight and food, the dizzying first phase of new romance may offer a temporary solution to overeating, says Susan Olson, Ph.D., a clinical psychologist and weight management specialist in Seattle. But like the phase itself, the effect on hunger is short-lived.

"Falling in love can help a woman who is an emotional eater," Dr. Olson says. "It's a distraction." A woman in the very first throes of love may be so absorbed with the relationship that food takes a backseat.

"Anticipation is a big appetite reducer," says Dr. Olson. If you're feeling butterflies in your stomach and can't think of much except Mr. Wonderful, you may be too excited to eat within your normal pattern.

Also, the sexual appetite of new love can overpower your physical appetite for food—but not for long. "As the relationship gets a little more comfortable, the sensuality of food can in fact be part of the thrill of a new partner," Dr. Olson says.

"All of the senses are heightened: Everything looks beautiful, you notice flowers, rain is wonderful, and sharing and enjoying food is part of that sensate experience."

"Being overweight in America now is a problem from the chin up, not the chin down," says Dr. McBarron.

Protecting Yourself with Fat

Maybe you can never be too thin or too rich, but some women can never be too fat. For them, fat serves as a kind of shield against the stresses and disappointments of life.

"If I'm fat and you don't like me, I can think it's because you're prejudiced against fat people," says Dr. McBarron. "If I lose weight and you still don't like me, then I can't blame it on my fat. So fat can be protective, mentally as well as physically."

That protection can also convey a certain image, says

Typecast Your Eating Trouble

Overeaters who fuel up because of feelings fall into five types, says Cynthia G. Last, Ph.D., author of *The Five Reasons Why We Overeat*. Identifying your type (most of us are combinations) takes you halfway to victory.

Impulse eater. You eat while standing up, talking on the phone, or watching TV, but you don't pay attention to how much you're eating.

Type fix: Eat at specific times and places; don't do anything else.

Hedonist. You treat food as pleasure or entertainment, but you gravitate toward high-fat, high-sugar foods. Taste is everything.

Type fix: Turn to alternatives. Get taste appeal from low-fat, low-cal choices like chocolate frozen ice pops instead of chocolate mousse.

Laurie L. Friedman, Ph.D., deputy director of Johns Hopkins Weight Management Center in Baltimore. "Some women feel that their size commands a certain kind of respect or that it can be intimidating," she says. Without the added weight, the women think they don't have that extra impact.

Women, especially those who have been overweight for long periods, may also use body size to avoid sexual involvement. "Women may get more attention from men if they lose weight, and for some, that attention is unwanted. It can be a bit scary," says Dr. Friedman.

Women have to realize that their fat serves a psychological purpose, says Dr. Last. Until they do, they'll never be able to control their eating. And if they do manage to

Stress reducer. You use food to relax when you're anxious or tense, but pressure or worry drives you to calorie-dense munchies like candy and potato chips.

Type fix: Defuse your mood with deep breathing, yoga, or exercise.

Avoider: You use food as a buffer against unpleasant situations or childhood trauma.

Type fix: Identify your real problems (unhealthy relationship? abusive boss or husband?) and develop problem-solving and assertiveness skills to handle them.

Energizer: You turn to food for a mood lift, resulting in weight gain. Your self-esteem drops and the cycle begins again.

Type fix: Fight a negative mindset with positive thoughts. Browse the "self-help" section in bookstores for ways to pulverize pessimism.

lose weight by focusing on external factors, like "bad" foods or poor eating habits, she says, this lack of awareness practically ensures that the pounds will return.

"It isn't so much what you eat that's important," Dr. Last says, "but what's really leading to overeating: emotions."

Understand Your Emotional Triggers

Key to gaining control over your weight is understanding what triggers your overeating.

Here are some tips to get you started.

Do the write thing. Keep paper and a pen next to the refrigerator. "Every time you find yourself there apart from mealtimes, think about what's going on and write it down," says Dr. Last. "Did you just argue with your husband? Are the kids screaming?" Eventually, you'll see a pattern. For example: "I eat every time I'm tense about the kids."

Make the refrigerator ring. Put a bell on the refrigerator door. It acts like an alarm clock for women who eat in the middle of the night or forage unthinkingly in the fridge.

Take time out. When stress, boredom, or the blues propel you toward that pint of rum raisin, give yourself time to take control. Cravings often pass within a short time, so set a cooking timer for 10 to 20 minutes and then decide whether you still want to eat, says Amy Joye Lund, R.D., nutrition specialist at the University of South Carolina's Weight Management Center in Charleston.

Outplan your appetite. For many women, overeating comes at the end of the workday, when they're home alone in front of the TV. So don't go there, says Lund. "Plan distractions for the times when you overeat." Take a walk or a shower, clean out a closet—do any nonfood activity that breaks the emotional eating routine. Plan to eat all your meals at the kitchen table, to remove the association between watching television and eating, Lund suggests.

Unlock your food prison. Allow yourself the occasional treat to avoid feelings of deprivation, says Dr. Schwartz. At her Yale weight center, clients who are going to a wed-

She Followed Her Own Rules

It's when she's happy—not stressed or bored—that Marlene Pixley encounters eating pitfalls. For more than 23 years, this 5-foot-3-inch homemaker has remained at 120 pounds, down from 152. Here's her secret.

"I do my emotional eating when life is good. I went through a divorce 13 years ago and lost weight. When someone in my life dies, I lose weight. So when things are on an even keel, I have to be careful.

"I used to be an evening TV snacker. There was always a bowl of jelly beans next to my chair, or soft cookies, or some cake. So my rule is, no food within easy reach while I watch TV. I don't even get satisfaction from the food because I'm not paying attention.

"Another rule is not eating in my car. I used to buy doughnuts and eat half of them on the way home. I don't deprive myself, though. In social situations or in a restaurant, I'll have the pie or cake (or doughnuts). I know myself well enough to know what rules I need, so I control my emotions ahead of time by making a conscious decision not to do this or that.

"My rules are mine. I give myself the flexibility to change them when I want to so that I don't feel like I've defeated myself if I break them. They help me set the stage for success."

ding, for example, are encouraged to have a piece of cake; it prevents overeating later.

Cut yourself some slack. Emotional eaters often have an all-or-nothing approach to weight loss, says Lund. If they eat a single cookie, they may think, "Well, I blew the day already; I might as well keep going." Keep it in perspective. "Look at that one instance in the context of the rest of the day or the rest of the week and realize how well you actually did. You might not have been perfect, but you weren't a total failure."

Stop feeling like a failure. Feeling like a failure when you eat unhealthfully is part of a common downward spiral in emotional eaters, Lund says. "A woman might have a burger and fries for lunch and come home feeling guilty for not having done the 'right thing.' Then she feels like she has lost control, so she inhales a dozen Oreos and feels even worse. A woman in this situation needs to remind herself that no one is perfect."

Setting a specific goal related to the behavior that is upsetting her can help, says Lund. "The goal should be reasonable, without the expectation of perfection. For example, if she has been eating burgers and fries almost every day, she should set a goal to limit burgers and fries to two times a week. Once she meets the goal or sees improvement, she may feel less like a failure."

To Change Eating Habits, Change Emotions

The key, then, is changing your emotional reactions to food, says Fugen Neziroglu, Ph.D., senior clinical director of the Bio-Behavioral Institute in Great Neck, New York.

Dr. Neziroglu uses cognitive therapy, which involves the patient and therapist in an active, goal-oriented approach to solving a specific problem, to help women identify erroneous thoughts or beliefs that may trigger undesirable eating.

So if your boss yells at you and you head for the vending machine, what's really going on?

Maybe you feel rejected, says Dr. Neziroglu. "You might say to yourself, 'I'm worthless; everyone is more competent than me,' and turn to food to avoid the feeling. That's the way you interpret the situation."

Instead, first try to understand your target trigger. Before you put any money in that vending machine, ask yourself: What just happened? What messages am I sending myself about the situation? What am I feeling?

Then challenge yourself. What thought or belief are you holding on to that may be false? Are you really incompetent, or is the boss just making you feel that way? Does the boss yell only at you, or does she yell at most of the staff? List all the areas in which you feel you are competent and all the people your boss yells at, then replay the scene in your mind, suggests Dr. Neziroglu. Now how do you feel?

By making the connection between emotions and food, says Dr. Neziroglu, you can "learn to gain control over the food rather than letting your addiction to food control you."

Eating Well to Lose

We are a generation of women on the go. From the minute our eyes open in the morning to the moment we gratefully let our heads sink onto the pillow at night, we are racing against time. Between commuting and chauffeuring our kids, we spend 64 minutes a day in the car. At noon, we do everything *but* stop for lunch, squeezing in the dry cleaner, bank, and post office during our average 36-minute lunch "hour."

After work, we hit the grocery store, one of our least favorite errands, sprinting through like a track star, grabbing for milk, bread, and something—*anything*—for dinner. Twenty-four minutes later, we're back in the minivan, wondering why we didn't just order pizza.

The result of our hurry-up lifestyle? Our rapidly expanding waistlines.

"We have worked very hard, practically since we were teenagers," says Irene O'Shaughnessy, M.D., associate professor of medicine at the Medical College of Wisconsin in Milwaukee. "We went to college. We shot for the sky professionally. Now we have families. Understandably, we've started looking for shortcuts, and often those shortcuts involve food."

Breakfast is a cup of coffee. We wolf down lunch at our desks. By the time dinner rolls around, we're famished and exhausted. No wonder we often choose the path of least resistance: fast food, Chinese takeout, or "home meal replacements" from the supermarket.

What we save in time, we gain in weight. We not only eat too much fat, sodium, and sugar but also deprive our bodies of the fiber, lean protein, fruits, and vegetables that they need to thrive and stay slim.

But eating a healthy diet doesn't require a Martha Stewart in the kitchen. "No one is saying that women need to start baking bread from scratch again," says Dr. O'Shaughnessy.

Nor does it mean a deprivation diet, dining on celery sticks, cottage cheese, and diet soda until we reach our goal weight. We simply need to make healthy eating a priority in our lives so we can enjoy satisfying meals that include not only food good for us but food that's just plain good.

Never Feel Hungry Again

After starving ourselves on diet after diet, we're ready to take Scarlett O'Hara's desperate vow as our own: "As God as my witness, I'll never be hungry again."

We don't have to be hungry. Losing weight safely and permanently doesn't require starvation diets, grapefruit diets, cabbage soup diets, bacon-and-egg diets, or any other type of "diet." In fact, weight-loss experts hate the idea of diets because going on a diet implies that one day we'll go off our diet and return to the same eating habits that contributed to our weight problem in the first place.

"I don't want women to feel hungry. I want them to eat when they feel hungry," says Gail Curtis, a certified physician assistant, assistant professor, and director of the weight management program at Wake Forest University Baptist Medical Center in Winston-Salem, North Carolina.

So think long-term—changing your lifestyle and eating patterns so you can keep the weight off forever. "You won't have rapid weight loss by eating right and exercising— maybe just a pound a week—but you'll develop habits that are permanent," say Katherine Chauncey, R.D., Ph.D., assistant professor and nutritionist at Texas Tech University Health Sciences Center in Lubbock.

And if you lose weight safely and slowly through better food choices, you shouldn't get those ravenous, I-have-to-eat-everything-in-the-cupboard feelings. Here's how to start.

Don't Put This in Your Pantry

Dietitians have stopped labeling foods as "good" or "bad," saying you can eat anything in small quantities. But even they make an exception for trigger foods—items that tempt you to eat far more than you intended, leading to a vicious cycle of disappointment and overeating. If you can't control how much you eat of a particular food, keep it out of your pantry. Nutritionists recommend barring the following items from the kitchen.

Treats for the kids. "If you have potato chips and cookies in the house for your kids, you're going to eat them, too," warns Laura Molseed, R.D., outpatient nutrition coordinator at the University of Pittsburgh Medical Center. Consider this a chance to set a healthy example. "Kids do what Mom does," Molseed adds.

Make friends with fiber. If you get 25 to 35 grams a day, you'll find that the pounds come off more easily and stay off. In one study, people who ate at least 21 grams of fiber a day gained 8 fewer pounds over a 10-year period than those who ate fewer than 12 grams. Fiber not only fills you up on less but stays with you longer. And numerous studies suggest that it also reduces your risk of heart disease, cancer, and diabetes. Good sources include legumes, fruits, vegetables, and whole-grain pastas, cereals, and breads.

Lunch with protein. If pasta salad with a roll represents your typical lunch, add some lean meats or legumes. Research suggests that a high-protein lunch is more filling than a high-carbohydrate one and may also help you eat less at dinner. Add lean turkey breast to your bagel, sprinkle chickpeas on your salad, or toss a carton of low-fat yogurt into your brown bag.

Soft drinks. They add up to serious calories—a 12-ounce can of regular cola contains 152 calories. Drink water instead.

Alcohol. Beer, wine, and liquor contain 7 calories per gram, almost as much as fat. And your metabolism handles them like fat, storing them for later use. "Women who want to lose weight while continuing to drink alcohol will have a harder time getting the results they want," says Cyndi Reeser, R.D., lead nutritionist at the Lipid Research Clinic at George Washington University in Washington, D.C.

Foods for us, foods for our families. Don't cook two meals. You and your family should be eating the same healthy food. If your family rebels, tell them they're free to make something else.

Don't forget fats. This is a tricky one, because eating too much fat is one reason people become heavy. But women tend to focus on fat and fat alone, ignoring calories, portion size, and exercise in favor of counting grams of fat. The result? Frustration.

"I've rarely found a woman who could lose weight successfully by just watching grams of fat," says Dr. Chauncey. "Men could make it work, but women rarely could." Men need more calories to begin with, she says, so when they start reducing fat, they actually reduce their calories, thus creating a calorie deficit. Women, on the other hand, need fewer calories to begin with, and when they replace regular foods with fat-free counterparts, they don't reduce overall calories that much.

You need a certain amount of fat in your diet. Fat influences the taste and texture of foods and affects how full you feel. Plus, not all fats are "bad." You want to limit the saturated fats, which are found mainly in red meat and other animal products, like butter and whole milk. They're the culprit when it comes to artery-clogging cholesterol. Instead, plan that 25 percent of your calories come from monounsaturated and polyunsaturated fats, found in fish, olive oil, nuts, and seeds. Studies show that monounsaturated fats in particular may reduce your risk of heart disease. So sprinkle nuts and seeds on your salads. Add avocado to your sandwiches. Use olive oil instead of butter for cooking. Keep the portions small; regardless of whether the fat is saturated or unsaturated, it still packs 9 calories per gram, compared with 4 for carbohydrates and protein.

Eat Early, Eat Often

The best way to lose weight? Eating. It sounds like a catch-22, but many weight-loss experts say that women who want to lose weight need first to learn how to eat.

That means breakfast, lunch, and dinner, with a few healthy snacks to keep the edge off.

"Most of us need to replenish our body fuel every 3 to 4 hours," says Cindy Moore, R.D., director of nutrition therapy at the Cleveland Clinic Foundation and a spokesperson for the American Dietetic Association. "Eating regularly keeps your blood sugar at stable, healthy levels so you stay energized."

It also keeps you motivated to make healthy choices.

"When your blood sugar is low, your willpower is low," Moore says. "That's when you're inclined to eat sweets or foods that are high in fat, like a candy bar, when you're preparing dinner."

"Eating also raises the metabolic rate," adds Cyndi Reeser, R.D., lead nutritionist at the Lipid Research Clinic at George Washington University in Washington, D.C. Just the process of digestion, absorption, and metabolism requires more energy than doing nothing, but when you start dieting, your resting metabolic rate goes down because you're taking in fewer calories. "If you dramatically cut back on calories, your body thinks it's starving," she says, "so it won't burn as many calories while it's resting."

Healthy snacks can help; so can eating more-substantial meals, especially earlier in the day. "Women often eat too lightly during the day and too heavily at night," says Reeser. She suggests reducing calories moderately for best results.

You need to balance your eating throughout the day, dividing your total calories roughly into fourths: one-fourth each to breakfast, lunch, dinner, and snacks.

The changes don't need to come all at once. Think about your own eating habits and daily routine. Perhaps you could nibble on fruit instead of potato chips for your afternoon snack or munch some toast and cheese with your morning cappuccino. Maybe you could bring your lunch a few times a week or eschew the local trattoria in favor of a home-cooked meal Friday nights.

Pick one change, says Moore. Stick to it for 2 weeks until it becomes a habit. At the end of the 2 weeks, choose another small change, carefully maintaining your previous healthy eating habit.

Plan Those Meals

By 4:00 P.M. every day, 60 percent of us still have no idea what we're having for dinner. That's a trend we need to change; when we're hungry, tired, and clueless about our next meal, we get into trouble.

But start slowly. Excitedly deciding to make every recipe in your new low-fat cookbook is likely to leave you with a refrigeratorful of spoiling food, a pizza delivery boy on your doorstep, and a boatload of frustration. So experts recommend these tips.

Be realistic. When you consider the coming week's menu, ask yourself how often you'll be eating out, when you'll be carrying lunch, and how many nights you'll be able to prepare dinner from scratch, suggests Joan Hammeren, R.D., a registered dietitian at the University of Colorado Health Sciences Center's Weight Choice program in Denver. Plan your menus and your grocery list at the same time.

Keep it simple. Don't stress yourself out by agonizing over every detail of each meal, says Franca Alphin, R.D., administrative director of the Diet and Fitness Center at Duke University in Durham, North Carolina. Weekly menu planning can be as easy as jotting down a main dish, such as "Monday: chicken" or "Friday: pizza." Fill in the fruits, vegetables, and grains from your well-stocked pantry and freezer.

Go short, go long. None of us have time to hit the supermarket on a daily basis, but we hate monster shopping trips even more. As a compromise, Hammeren suggests making "short shops" once or twice a week to buy just what you need in terms of produce, lean meats, dairy, and lunch items. Save the staples for occasional "big shops."

Stock the nonperishables. During those "big shops," buy basics such as canned beans, quick brown rice, pasta, canned green chiles, couscous, low-sodium chicken broth, canned tomatoes, and other staples for on-the-fly weeknight dinners, Hammeren recommends. Keep your freezer stocked with frozen vegetables, including chopped onions and peppers and whole-grain breads.

What's the Deal with Water?

Diet programs advocate eight glasses of water daily because you need to stay well-hydrated. Your body is composed primarily of water, and you need to constantly flush out the old fluids and refresh yourself with new ones.

Caffeinated products, like coffee, tea, and cola, dehydrate you. So do alcohol and air travel. Drinking eight glasses of water gives you back the minimum your body needs.

When you don't drink enough water, you tend to be thirsty all the time. You may feel tired. If you keep well-hydrated, you'll feel more alert and energized. And if you feel better, you're more apt to be in control of other things—like your weight.

Expert consulted: Franca Alphin, R.D., administrative director, Diet and Fitness Center, Duke University, Durham, North Carolina

Make a list. Is there anything more frustrating than reaching into your cupboard for a quick supper of canned tomatoes and dried pasta, only to find that you used the last of them for veggie lasagna the other night? Post a running grocery list on your fridge or inside your organizer. When you're almost out of something, write it down, suggests Hammeren.

Cook in quantity. It's as easy to cook for 12 as it is for 6. Just double the recipe. Freeze enough for another meal and use leftovers for lunches, Hammeren adds.

Back to Basics

So you're planning your menus. What should they consist of?

Real food. Food that still bears some resemblance to its original state. This means fruits and vegetables, whole grains, beans, legumes, lean meats, water.

"Anytime you can eat a simple food, like a grilled chicken breast, it'll be lower in calories than fried chicken or chicken with a high-fat sauce," says Mary Martha Smoak, R.D., a registered dietitian at Wake Forest University Baptist Medical Center in Winston-Salem, North Carolina. Unprocessed foods also have more naturally occurring nutrients, including various vitamins, minerals, and fiber, and less added sodium, sugar, and fat.

Here's how to reorient your meals toward natural choices.

Drink water. Cold and calorie-free, water is your best friend in your lifestyle change. Choosing it over soda, sweetened fruit drinks, and sweetened tea, as often as you can, could let you lose up to 1 pound a week, says Dr. Chauncey.

It's not that you'll eat less—contrary to a common weight-loss myth, water doesn't fill you up. But you won't be adding extra calories from a nonfilling liquid either, says Smoak. Some women discover through food diaries that they can drink as many as 1,000 calories a day without feeling full from the liquid.

You'll also stay well-hydrated. "Women often drink too little water," Reeser says. "They forget the role that fluid balance plays in weight reduction and general health."

To liven up your eight daily glasses, have the water over ice with a twist of lemon or lime. Can't stand the chemical taste of tap water? Use filtered pitchers or splurge for bottled. Choose calorie-free carbonated waters for a fizzy treat, drink unsweetened herbal teas hot or cold, and dilute your favorite juice with water for a low-calorie thirst quencher.

Look for whole grains. By eating whole-grain breads, cereals, and pastas, you'll boost your fiber intake, filling your stomach while you trim calories. But remember, just because a bread isn't white doesn't mean it has a lot of fiber in it. Some brown breads, for example, get their hue from caramel coloring. Read food labels carefully. You want "whole grains" listed as one of the top ingredients, says Dr. O'Shaughnessy.

Other good sources include barley, whole wheat couscous, and brown and wild rice, says Moore. For noodle lovers, many supermarkets now carry whole wheat pasta. If your family is new to whole-grain pasta, start slowly. Mix one part whole-grain noodles to two parts regular, then up the whole-grain proportion as you become adjusted to the taste and higher fiber content.

Learn to love beans. High in protein, dried beans and legumes should be a staple in your diet. They're a meat substitute for vegetarians as well as a healthy complement to beef, chicken, and fish.

Filled with fiber, beans and lentils break down slowly in your body, keeping your stomach full longer and your blood sugar level stable, says Laura Molseed, R.D., outpatient nutrition coordinator at the University of Pittsburgh Medical Center. This sends a one-two knockout punch to temptation when the office pastry cart appears or you pass a vending machine.

Forget dried beans that need overnight soaking and 3 hours on the stove. Canned beans (rinse them to eliminate most of the sodium) go nicely in salads, spaghetti sauces, and casseroles. Dried lentils, on the other hand, do cook fast.

Finagle more fruits. Low in calories and high in nutrients, fruit qualifies as a dietary mainstay of many university weight management programs. Dr. Chauncey tells her patients to eat as much fruit as they want. It's healthy, and it keeps the hunger pangs at bay. But she cautions those with diabetes to check with their doctors before eating large portions of certain fruits.

Overnight Weight Loss?

The reason you weigh less in the morning—when all you've done for the past 8 hours is sleep—is because of your body's nightly rebalancing act. During the day, you're drinking. You're eating. And your body is slowly but surely metabolizing those calories. As it does this, you retain water because water is required to store fat and carbohydrates. At night, your body settles into a level of balance, and your kidneys are able to filter out any unnecessary fluids. This allows you to reach your lowest level of weight by early morning (after urinating).

Expert consulted: Pamela Peeke, M.D., assistant clinical professor of medicine, University of Maryland, Bethesda, and author of *Fight Fat after Forty*

If getting the recommended five a day sounds about as likely as your teenager awakening before noon on a Saturday, have faith (and follow these simple tips).

- Remember the saying "out of sight, out of mind"? That goes double for fruit. If you're lucky enough to be in the market for a new refrigerator, look for one with clear shelves and drawers so that you can see what's hiding behind the milk. Otherwise, post a list of just-purchased fruit on the refrigerator door or keep your fruit in a pretty bowl or basket on the counter.

  Apply the same principle at work. If you bring grapes for a snack, don't leave them to bruise in your briefcase or turn into gray glop in the refrigerator. Put them on your desk for mindful munching.

- For the best taste and prices on fresh produce, learn what's in season when. Somehow a cantaloupe in January just isn't going to have the same sweet-as-sugar taste as one eaten in July. You'll also save if you purchase just what you know you'll eat. Live alone? You don't need an entire box of clementines; just a few navel oranges will do nicely. Finally, don't forget about canned and frozen fruits. Look for fruits canned in light syrup or in their own juices; they're lower in calories.

Venerate veggies. Whether you like them steamed or stir-fried, roasted or raw, vegetables should be the mainstay on your plate. From the calcium in broccoli to the lycopene in tomatoes, vegetables contain vitamins, minerals, and phytonutrients essential to your health no matter what you weigh.

Like fruit, vegetables satisfy with minimal calories, providing about 3 grams of fiber per serving cooked or raw. To get more into your diet, stir chopped veggies into spaghetti sauce. Add sprouts or lettuce and tomato to sandwiches.

Eat yams for snacks (cook them quickly in the microwave). Look for packages of baby carrots, prewashed mixed greens, and ready-to-go salads.

"Buying already prepared vegetables may seem expensive, but if you eat them, they're worth it," says Suzanne W. Dixon, R.D., a research epidemiologist and registered dietitian at the Henry Ford Health System in Detroit.

Got milk? "Women do not drink enough milk," says Dr. O'Shaughnessy, who treats women for osteoporosis. "They're worried about the extra calories, and it's not as convenient as a diet soda from the office vending machine."

Yet milk may be a weight-loss catalyst.

When researchers followed women for 2 years, they discovered that those who ate fewer than 1,900 calories and consumed at least 1,000 milligrams of calcium daily—primarily from fat-free milk, yogurt, and regular cheese— lost 6 pounds of body fat. Women who took in fewer than 500 milligrams of calcium gained 2 to 3 pounds of body fat.

To get your daily calcium, try 1 cup of low-fat cottage cheese (400 milligrams), 8 ounces of fat-free milk (300 milligrams), 1 cup of low-fat yogurt (350 milligrams), and ½ cup of fat-free frozen yogurt (50 milligrams).

Break the Fast

Women, notorious breakfast skippers in the best of nutritional times, are even worse when trying to lose weight, says Molseed. In a misguided attempt to cut calories, we skip the first meal of the day—with disastrous consequences for our diets.

"It only ends up making you hungrier later," Molseed says. In contrast, when you start your day with a small meal, you may be less likely to overeat at later meals because you won't feel so ravenous, says Hammeren.

For a morning meal that keeps you going until lunch, combine carbohydrates like oatmeal, high-fiber cold cereal, or whole wheat bread with lean protein like low-fat milk, yogurt, or scrambled eggs made with egg substitute, suggests Hammeren.

Breakfast is also the perfect meal to begin sneaking in servings of fruit, says Alphin. Sprinkle fresh or frozen blueberries over cereal, stir raisins into oatmeal, or mix thawed frozen strawberries into yogurt.

If you can't remember the last time your day started with more than a low-fat latte to go, give these tips a try.

Say hello to cereal. With fat-free milk, cereal is low-fat and low-fuss. Check the nutrition information before you buy; you want a cereal with no more than 14 grams of sugar per serving and at least 7 grams of fiber. "If you eat something very sweet at breakfast, you'll set yourself up for more sweets later when your blood sugar crashes," Alphin says. If you can't live without Cap'n Crunch, mix half with a high-fiber variety like Post Raisin Bran or Kellogg's All-Bran.

Think liquid. No time to sit and eat? Take it with you. Blend 1 cup fat-free milk with half a frozen banana, 1 teaspoon sugar, 1 cup frozen strawberries, and enough soy powder to equal 7 grams of protein for a sweet, creamy smoothie.

Get toasted. Start your day right with the protein–carb combo of peanut butter or low-fat cream cheese on a slice of whole wheat toast, an English muffin, or half a bagel.

Go portable. Stock your fridge with hard-cooked eggs, cartons of yogurt, and sliced cheese that you can slap on some bread and take with you for breakfast on the run. If you have an extra few minutes, stir ¼ cup of Grape-Nuts cereal into yogurt for extra crunch and fiber.

Remember old favorites. On a chilly morning, oatmeal makes a comforting, high-fiber breakfast. Combine ½ cup oats with 1 cup fat-free milk, 1 apple (chopped and un-peeled), 2 tablespoons wheat germ, and 2 teaspoons brown sugar. Cook according to the directions on the package of oatmeal.

Beat the clock. If the smell of scrambled eggs in the morning makes you burrow under the bedcovers, skip breakfast in favor of brunch. Before the clock strikes noon, eat a piece of fruit, a slice of toast, a stick of string cheese, or some low-fat yogurt, says Hammeren.

Eat lightly at night. Not hungry in the morning? Eat less in the evening. "It's best to curb food intake at night, when metabolism slows," Reeser says. "Do whatever it takes to keep your hands busy. Make crafts. Write. If you must go to bed to avoid eating, go to bed. You'll be hungrier in the morning." Then you can eat that good-for-you breakfast.

Go for Low Energy Density

For Barbara Rolls, Ph.D., coauthor of *Volumetrics: Feel Full on Fewer Calories*, the key to losing weight isn't just calories or grams of fat but also "energy density." Basically, energy density is affected by how much water a food contains. The higher the water content, the lower the energy density. The lower the energy density, the fuller you'll feel on fewer calories.

Also, the more fat in a food, the higher its energy density because fat packs a lot of calories into a small amount of food, says Dr. Rolls, who is also the Guthrie Chair of Nutrition at Pennsylvania State University in University Park.

Dry and high in fat, potato chips qualify as high energy-density food, while broth-based vegetable soup is low, helped by the high water content of the broth and the vegetables.

Even if you've never heard of the concept, energy density influences how much you eat. "Day after day, people tend to eat a constant weight or volume of food because they've learned how much usually satisfies them," Dr. Rolls says. For instance, you're going to eat three slices of pizza, whether it has sausage or vegetables on it. But if you ordered the one with vegetables, you'd be just as full on far fewer calories. Since you're going to be eating the same amount, she says, make sure that what you're eating is low energy density so that it will also be low in calories.

Energy density can also trip you up when you're trying to lose weight. "When women diet, they start eating tiny

Large Portions, Low Calories

It's a dieter's dream: Eat a lot to lose a lot. You can do that when your foods have a low calorie density. The more fat a food contains, the more calorie dense it is. Oil, for example, is all fat, so it tops the calorie density list. But a whole cup of raw spinach, with virtually no fat, has a very low calorie density.

If you want the most volume of food that will still let you lose weight, look for items like these, which give you large portions with few calories.

Food	Calories per Serving	Calories per Gram
Grilled chicken (6 oz)	270	1.5
Broiled flounder (6 oz)	200	1.2
Baked potato with skin (7 oz)	220	1.1
Low-fat fruit yogurt (8 oz)	243	1.0
One apple (medium)	81	0.6
One raw carrot (large)	30	0.4
Cooked broccoli (½ cup)	22	0.3
Raw spinach (1 cup)	6	0.2

portions," Dr. Rolls says. "They haven't learned that it's important to fill their plates for visual and physical reasons." Those tiny portions will just leave you aching for more food. When you choose foods low in energy density, however, such as strawberries or spinach, you can eat enough to fill you up yet not worry about high calories, she says.

Here's how you can lower the energy density of your meals.

Add extra vegetables to entrées. Instead of a cup of pasta with ½ cup of Alfredo sauce, toss 1 cup of cooked pasta with tomatoes, summer squash, mushrooms, broccoli, olive oil, Parmesan cheese, and herbs. For the same calories, you'll be able to eat 3½ cups of pasta primavera, versus 1½ cups of the Alfredo. Also try adding grapes and apples to chicken salad or piling veggies on pizza.

Slurp soup. With their high water content, broth-based soups are the queens of low-energy-density foods. When Dr. Rolls served women soup for lunch, they ate fewer

What's a Portion?

Portion control can be a guessing game if you can't estimate serving sizes. Here are some easy equivalents.

This much ...	is the size of ...
1½ oz cheese	a pair of dice
1 cup vegetables	your fist
1 medium apple	a baseball
½ cup pasta, rice, or potatoes	a scoop of ice cream
1 cup dry cereal	a large handful
3 oz lean meat	a deck of cards

calories at that meal and didn't make up for them at dinner, compared with those who dined on an equally caloric casserole accompanied by a glass of water. Take advantage of these effects when you're eating out, by ordering broth-based (not cream) soup as an appetizer.

Start with salad. An appetizer salad of leafy greens will take the edge off your appetite before your higher-calorie entrée arrives. To keep the meal's energy density down, use less regular dressing or opt for fat-free dressing instead.

Choose fresh fruits over dried. If you have trouble eating fresh produce before it spoils, dried fruits are the perfect answer. But their high energy density means that a little box of raisins goes a long way calorie-wise. When you're starving at 3:00 P.M., 2 cups of grapes are more filling than ¼ cup of raisins, with the same number of calories.

Calories Do Count

You've trimmed the fat in your breakfasts, lunches, and dinners. You're eating foods with low energy density. You're snacking on fruits and veggies. But the pounds still aren't melting away. Perhaps it's time to look at your overall calories.

"With many women who are struggling to lose weight, it's not so much the makeup of their meals but how much they're eating," says Hammeren.

Trim 200 to 500 calories each day—the equivalent of a couple of sodas and a piece of cheesecake. Just be sure that your overall calorie count doesn't drop below 1,200, or you'll miss out on vital nutrients, says Curtis.

Add enough exercise to burn another 250 calories daily—about 45 minutes of brisk walking—and you'll lose roughly 1 to 2 pounds a week. It sounds like slow going, but it works.

"We understand you want to lose the weight yesterday," says Curtis. "But you have to remember that you didn't gain it yesterday."

To cut calories, you don't need to eliminate foods; just control portion sizes.

But what is a portion, anyway? "Some people seem to think that a portion is whatever they eat or whatever they're served," Smoak says. The answer is far more precise. For instance, 1 cup of leafy raw vegetables (such as spinach or romaine lettuce), ½ cup of cooked or raw veggies (such as carrots or cooked spinach), and ½ cup of cooked legumes all qualify as a portion of vegetables.

A serving of fruit? That would be ¾ cup of juice—not the tumblerful of orange drink that you down each morning. The same goes for bagels. Halve that hunk of boiled bread to get one serving, according to the USDA.

Make Time for Meals

As a busy mom of two children, Alayne Gunto rarely sat down to eat, especially when she was in the middle of a task. "If I was cleaning house, I never stopped long enough for a meal," says Alayne, who lives in Moundsville, West Virginia. "I'd grab a handful of potato chips. I never ate breakfast. By 11:00 A.M., I'd be starving. But I wouldn't eat lunch either; I'd just snatch crackers or a peanut butter and jelly sandwich."

Her nonstop habits had serious consequences. When she joined TOPS in 1996, Alayne weighed 235 pounds.

Today, she's 100 pounds slimmer. Her advice on controlling an out-of-control appetite? Eat regular meals, and don't leave home without healthy snacks and condiments.

"I had to learn to eat three meals a day," Alayne says. Breakfast was the biggest challenge. She found

But even dietitians admit that measuring food gets tedious fast. So they recommend trying these shortcuts.

Test yourself. Get out your favorite cereal bowl, coffee cup, and juice glass. Fill them with the quantity of food and drinks that you normally have. Then pour their contents into measuring cups. How does your morning bowl of cereal compare with the recommended serving size on the packages? How many servings are you actually eating? If you discover that you're drinking 1½ cups of apple juice every morning, trade half those liquid calories for an apple. You'll get more stomach-filling fiber, and your blood sugar level will be stabler than if you just drank the juice alone.

Watch proportions. For a well-balanced meal that supports your weight loss, divide your dinner plate into quarters. Allocate one-quarter for lean protein, one-half for

that the best time for her morning meal was after her children left for school and her husband went to work. "Some days, it's oatmeal or raisin bran; other days, I'll have half a bagel or English muffin and some fruit. That's usually enough to tide me over until lunchtime," Alayne says.

Alayne's healthy new habits have carried over to other meals. She takes time for a light lunch, preparing herself a salad or tuna sandwich. And when she's on the go, she travels prepared, carrying pretzels or fruit with her. Should she end up at a restaurant or fast-food joint, she's ready for that, too, with packets of fat-free dressing and fat-free butter spray for seasoning bread, steamed veggies, or popcorn.

vegetables or fruits, and one-quarter for grains. "Women overcarb it," says Pamela Peeke, M.D., assistant clinical professor of medicine at the University of Maryland in Bethesda and author of *Fight Fat after Forty*. "Men over-protein it. They eat a hunk of steak. We eat a hunk of bagel." As you age, your metabolism slows down, and you no longer need all the energy contained in starchy foods such as pasta, rice, potatoes, and breads, Dr. Peeke says. Treat carbohydrates like a treat, especially at dinnertime, basing your meals on veggies and fruit instead.

Use smaller dishes. Your petite plates and bowls will look satisfying and full even with smaller portions.

Check your temptations. You can never eat too many fruits and vegetables, but it's easy to overdo other luscious foods. If you suspect that you're overeating certain foods, grab your measuring cup and find out. You don't have to give up the blueberry muffin from the neighborhood bakery, but you should know how many servings it consti-tutes and how many calories and grams of fat it con-tributes to your day. Then you can occasionally work it into your food plan.

Don't eat out of containers. "I find it very hard to mon-itor how many chips I've eaten when I'm just dipping my hand into the bag," Reeser admits. So pour out a portion, seal the package, and put it away.

Indulge Yourself

Chocolate chip cookie dough. Sour cream and onion potato chips. Mashed potatoes with real butter. Whether your tastes tend toward sweet, sour, or salty, you know you have culinary indulgences that you can't live without, no matter how many pounds you want to lose.

And you don't have to. "If you really want a Snickers bar every day, then plan it in," Alphin says.

There will be trade-offs, however. You may not be able to eat both the Snickers bar and the potato chips every day, or an entire pint of ice cream at one sitting. But you don't need to deny yourself foods that you genuinely relish in the name of weight loss. Such a rigid approach to eating would make you feel deprived and rebellious. So if you're eating nothing but spinach salad for a week straight, sooner or later you're going to have a Fritos binge, blindly munching chip after chip until nothing is left but the salt that you're licking off your fingers.

Instead, incorporate small, edible pleasures into each day. "Food should be pleasurable," says Judith S. Stern, R.D., Sc.D., professor of nutrition and internal medicine at the University of California, Davis. "We all want to eat and enjoy it, but no one wants her life to be ruled by it."

So try this.

Indulge in only what you love. When Alphin recommends changes to her patients' eating habits, she often hears, "I never really liked that anyhow." If a sliver of cheesecake is what makes your heart beat faster, don't waste those calories on kettle-cooked potato chips.

Time your treats. Give in to your sweet cravings when you're least likely to overeat, Dr. Stern advises. If a week without ice cream is like Christmas without Santa, order it in small amounts for dessert when you're dining at a restaurant. That way, you won't be standing in front of your refrigerator, scooping it out of the carton.

Buy small quantities. When we purchase jumbo packages, we end up eating jumbo-size portions. Researchers at the University of Illinois at Urbana–Champaign found that people ate between 7 and 43 percent more food when serving themselves from larger containers. That's not a problem if you're buying a bushel of apples, but it will be if your grocery cart is stuffed with family-size bags of cheese doodles. Purchase single-serving packages of sweet or salty treats. If it's ice cream you love, buy pints or ice cream bars rather than half-gallons.

Make it a ritual. Create a ceremony to revel in your favorite food pleasures. Serve ice cream in ramekins, with delicate spoons, after dinner. Use your best china for french fries. You'll eat more slowly and enjoy every bite.

Consider substitutes. Save fat and calories by looking for lighter versions of food luxuries. Choose baked tortilla chips instead of fried, sorbet over full-fat ice cream, diet soda instead of regular. Just don't devour the entire package, thinking that "fat-free" means "calorie-free." Many fat-free items are just as high in sugar and calories as their regular counterparts. "Once you eat three servings of a fat-free item, it's no longer fat-free," says Reeser.

Go for the real thing. Substitutes don't always satisfy. If you hate the taste of low-fat cheese, for example, buy the real stuff and eat it in small, flavorful quantities that give you as much taste per calorie as possible. When you control your portion size, no food is forbidden indefinitely, says Hammeren.

How Activity Burns Fat

W hy spend hundreds of dollars on expensive exercise equipment when you can get the same calorie burn with a broom, a dustpan, and a warren of dust bunnies?

That's right. Housework burns fat. Until recently, it seemed that the only way to solve the *burn more calories* part of the weight-loss equation was to sweat it out at the gym for an hour or so several times a week. Not so. Research shows that moderate activity can burn fat just as efficiently as a structured exercise program.

So what exactly qualifies as moderate-intensity activity?

On the effort scale, moderate would rate the equivalent of a brisk walk. That's about as fast as you might walk if you were late for an appointment or trying to catch a bus, says Bess H. Marcus, Ph.D., associate professor of psychiatry and human behavior at the Brown University Center for Behavioral and Preventive Medicine in Providence, Rhode Island. It's not a stroll through the mall.

One study, called Project Active, conducted at the Cooper Institute for Aerobics Research in Dallas, compared two ways of getting 235 sedentary men and women moving. Half the participants were instructed to work out in a gym for 30 minutes at least three times a week. The other half met one night a week in small groups to discuss ways to integrate physical activity into their lives.

Instead of going to the gym, the lifestyle group found ways to use the stairs more often, walk farther to restrooms, and generally make life a little more labor intensive. "People got real creative about how to work more activity into their lives. Physical activity was suddenly on their radar screen," says Dr. Marcus, who was one of the coauthors of the study.

After just 6 months, both groups had comparable increases in physical activity, using up about 150 extra calories a day. That's the equivalent of about 30 minutes of moderate-intensity activity—all you need to start burning fat.

Every Step Counts

Instead of thinking of exercise as pain and sweat, think of it as your body in motion—any kind of motion. Or to put it another way: The more you move your arms and legs, the more calories you burn. The more you sit or lie still, the fewer calories you burn.

The problem is, we're doing too much sitting and too little moving. Blame our harried schedules or the conveniences of modern technology. With the click of a switch, we can open a garage door, change the channel on the TV, or go shopping all over the globe. All in all, fewer than one in four of us gets the 30 minutes of daily activity recommended by health experts. That's a lot of unspent calories.

According to a study from the United Kingdom, people there burn about 800 fewer calories per day than they did

Burnin' Calories

If you are a 150-pound woman, how long does it take to burn 150 more calories a day? That depends on what you do. (If you weigh more, it may take less intensity to burn the same amount of calories.)

Activity	Time
Ironing	59 minutes
Cooking	48 minutes
Washing and waxing a car	45–60 minutes
Playing volleyball	45 minutes
Strolling through the mall	44 minutes
Grocery shopping	36 minutes
Doing yoga	36 minutes
Vacuuming	34 minutes
Playing horseshoes	33 minutes
Gardening	30–45 minutes
Bicycling leisurely	5 miles in 30 minutes
Brisk walking	30 minutes
Dancing fast	30 minutes
Pushing a stroller	30 minutes
Raking leaves	30 minutes
Mowing with a power push mower	29 minutes
Inline skating leisurely	26 minutes
Stacking firewood	25 minutes
Bowling	23 minutes
Housecleaning	21 minutes
Scrubbing floors	20 minutes
Swimming	19 minutes
Climbing stairs	15 minutes
Shoveling snow	15 minutes

in 1970, mostly because of automation and labor-saving devices. It's the same story on this side of the Atlantic.

"Physical activity has been pushed out of our lives," says Miriam Nelson, Ph.D., associate chief of the Human Physiology Laboratory at the Jean Mayer USDA Human Nutrition Research Center on Aging at Tufts University in Boston and author of *Strong Women Stay Slim*. "It is no longer a part of our social fabric. This means we have to choose ways to work activity back into our lives. We have

A Bad Habit Pays Off

You call it fidgeting. Researchers know it as NEAT (nonexercise activity thermogenesis). Either way, unconscious movements like changing posture, tapping your feet, and moving around burn excess calories.

For 2 months, researchers at the Mayo Clinic in Rochester, Minnesota, fed 16 normal-weight people an extra 1,000 calories a day—the caloric equivalent of two Big Macs. Then they tracked whether the calories were burned or stored as fat or lean tissue.

The amount of weight the participants gained varied from 2 to 16 pounds. The reason for the difference: the number of calories burned through NEAT. While some people burned fewer than 100 calories a day, others burned nearly 700 calories.

The message from this study is an optimistic one: Every calorie you burn by moving around counts. And although NEAT is probably something you do unconsciously, researchers speculate that you may be able to train yourself to increase NEAT by using behavioral cues, such as putting music on while you're doing dishes and moving to the beat.

to consciously get up more, walk more, take the stairs more. Whenever possible, we need to seek out activity."

Most moderate-intensity activities—walking briskly, raking leaves, mowing the lawn with a push mower, or vacuuming—will burn 150 calories in about 30 minutes. So instead of just counting calories, also add up your minutes of activity each day. To lose weight and keep it off, you actually need about 60 minutes of activity a day, according to the latest research.

It doesn't make any difference if you do it all at once or break it up into smaller chunks of time. "Everything counts," says Barbara Moore, Ph.D., president of Shape Up America! in Washington, D.C.

Step up the intensity. Michelle Edwards, a health educator and certified personal trainer at the Cooper Institute, advises her clients to start by simply increasing the intensity of any physical activity that they're already doing. That can mean taking the stairs a little faster, choosing parking spots at the far end of the lot, or making wider arm circles when wiping off the kitchen counter. The idea is to put a little more effort into every activity in order to burn more calories.

Keep a diary. For the next few days, clock yourself every time you walk, clean, garden, climb a flight of stairs, or perform any other activity that involves moving the muscles in your arms and legs. At the end of the day, add up your active time. It helps create a vivid picture of how the minutes add up, explains Edwards. Once you do this, you'll probably find yourself thinking of all kinds of ways to add a few more minutes here and there throughout the day.

One of the keys to becoming more active is learning to identify opportunities in your day and taking advantage of them. "Five minutes here; ten minutes there. It all adds up," says Edwards.

It also helps to record how much time you spend sitting each day. Figure out ways to gradually reduce that amount.

Get a pedometer. If you want to get a clearer picture of the amount of physical activity you are doing in a day, record how many steps you take on an average day and then find ways to add more. Studies show that people who are active for 30 minutes each day accumulate about 10,000 steps, while the average person who works in an office typically takes about 2,000 to 4,000 steps a day. "A pedometer can be a very motivational tool, a way to self-monitor," says Edwards. "And we know from experience that people who self-monitor are more likely to reach their activity goals than people who do not."

Be prepared. Keep walking shoes in your car or desk so that you can walk whenever you have a few minutes, says Edwards.

Schedule it. We tend to keep our appointments, so make an appointment to exercise. You can start by scheduling exercise in the morning instead of later in the day, suggests Denise Bruner, M.D., president of the American Society of Bariatric Physicians and a physician practicing in Arlington, Virginia. "Women seem to be more successful in general if they put activity on the front end of the day, versus the end of the day, when either work-related issues or home issues can end up taking precedence over exercise time," she says.

Working Activity In at Work

A hundred years ago, the average woman burned about 50 percent more calories a day. There was no need to worry about making sure you moved your body enough. Movement was built into each and every day.

"Basically, at the turn of the 20th century, something like 85 percent of our workforce worked in agriculture-related jobs," says Dr. Moore. "They were very physically demanding. In today's information-based society, so much of the work we do requires sitting and only sitting."

Besides sleeping, a lot of us spend the biggest chunk of our time at work. If you can work in three 10-minute walks over the course of your day, you'll burn an extra 150 calories. In a year, that adds up to more than 10 pounds of fat-burning calories. Here's how you can work in a workout.

Park on the outskirts. As in most cities, parking is scarce in Boston. Dr. Nelson ends up parking about eight blocks from her office each day. But instead of taking the university-provided shuttle, she walks the rest of the way. "I get an 8-minute walk every morning and afternoon. Then I add in a little bit here and there, and before you know it, I've burned a fair number of calories," she says.

No-Sweat Calorie Burning

A sauna can do more than help you relax, improve circulation, and relieve tension and anxiety. It can help you burn calories.

When you take a sauna, the heat hastens circulation, brings bloodflow to the skin, and stimulates sweating. While you're sitting back taking in the heat, the increased circulation and sweat response burn extra calories. During a half-hour sauna, you can expect to lose roughly 1 to 2 pounds of fluid. Each pound of sweat loss represents 263 calories of dissipated heat.

Note: If you are pregnant or if you have diabetes, multiple sclerosis, or high or low blood pressure, seek the advice of your physician before using a sauna.

Change your bus stop. If you ride public transportation, you probably already do a fair amount of walking. If you want to add a few more steps to your day, Dr. Moore recommends getting off your mode of transit a few stops early.

Take advantage of the speakerphone. Walk around or do stretches while you're on the phone, says Dr. Moore. Standing burns about 30 percent more calories than sitting.

Seek out the stairs instead of the elevator. "Buildings are designed so that the elevator is prominent and the stairs are not," says Dr. Moore. Stairways are tucked away in the far corners of the building and may not seem accessible. Seek them out. "Every opportunity should be seized to take a few steps." If you work in a high-rise, get off the elevator a few floors early and take the stairs the rest of the way. Add more floors as you build stamina.

Schedule a mobile meeting. Instead of sitting in a conference room and meeting over a cup of coffee, schedule a walking meeting, says Edwards.

Take the long way around. Whenever you're walking somewhere, take the long route, whether you're headed to the mail room or the conference room, says Dr. Nelson. Remember, every extra minute of walking burns about 5 calories.

Use the restroom on another floor. If you work in a one-story building, use the restroom farthest away from your desk, suggests Dr. Moore.

Set an activity timer. Program your computer or watch to remind you to take a brief walk, says Dr. Marcus. Some of the people in the Project Active study set their watches to go off each hour to remind them to take a 5-minute walk. At the end of the workday, they had accumulated 30 to 40 minutes of activity.

Order out. Build activity into your lunch hour. Instead of using the entire hour or half-hour to eat, save at least

10 minutes for a brisk walk. Or you could try ordering your lunch from a restaurant that's six blocks away, instead of one that's right around the corner, and then walk to get it, says Dr. Nelson.

Never take the escalator down. No, you don't burn as many calories walking down the steps as you do going up, but it's still an opportunity to move those muscles, says Dr. Moore. To boost your burn, swing your arms as you're walking down the stairs or downhill.

Activate Your Life Every Day

Our harried home lives often feel anything but inactive. We're constantly on the go, from the moment our feet hit the floor in the morning until the last chore is done at night. Who has time to squeeze one more thing onto their to-do list? The good news is that you don't have to do more; you just need to do it differently. You can find hidden opportunities for exercise simply by changing your approach to everyday chores and errands.

Don't let things pile up when you pick up. Eliminate using the bottom stairs as a holding area for stuff that needs to go on another floor, says Dr. Moore. Walk up and down the stairs every time you come across something that needs to be put away.

Walk and talk. Don't settle into your favorite chair for a good, long tête-à-tête when your best friend calls. Take advantage of the mobility you get using the cordless phone. Walk around, put away odds and ends, or go up and down the stairs while you talk.

Be an active captive. From women in the Project Active study, researchers heard a lot about having to take their kids places. "Think if there is some way for *you* to get more activity while you're a captive at your child's activities," says Dr. Marcus. Walk around the soccer field while

Is Thriller TV a Calorie-Burner?

Sorry—you burn the same number of calories watching a heart-racing Stephen King thriller as you do enjoying a pleasant sitcom, according to researchers at the University of Newcastle on Tyne in England. Sitting is sitting, it turns out.

Even so, watching TV doesn't have to be a totally listless experience, says Michelle Edwards, a health educator and certified personal trainer at the Cooper Institute for Aerobics Research in Dallas.

Instead of staying put during commercials, stand up and walk in place, do jumping jacks, skip rope, or just dance, says Edwards. The average adult watches 22 hours of TV a week. Considering that an hour-long prime-time drama has about 20 minutes of commercials, that adds up to a whopping 440 minutes of potential activity per week. Still think you don't have time to exercise?

watching the game. Take a walk around the block during the half-hour piano lesson.

Get lean while you clean. We're spending about 18 hours a week doing housework—half the time that our mothers spent. "I always recommend that people do housework to boost their activity level," says Dr. Moore. We're not suggesting that you step back into the days of domestic drudgery, but when you do cleaning, use large, exaggerated movements, and you'll burn more calories.

Do your own yard work. No more hiring a neighborhood kid to rake leaves or cut grass. Doing an hour of yard work a week burns about 300 extra calories. But don't use a power mower. "If you do, you won't burn 300 calories of your fat. You'll burn gasoline instead," says Dr. Moore.

Tote more groceries. It seems much more efficient to try to lug every single bag of groceries into the house in one trip. But you can burn more calories if you make multiple trips and bring the bags in one at a time, says Dr. Moore.

Go back to basics. Find places in your day where you can do a task in a more manual way, says Dr. Nelson. Get out the hose and wash your car yourself instead of taking it to the car wash. Lose your remote control and get up off the couch to switch channels. Walk to the store for a gallon of milk.

PART THREE

The Minor Keys of Success

Exercise as an Option

Now, hold on a minute! Just because you can get a great calorie burn from all your daily activities doesn't mean that regular exercise isn't a good idea.

If you put aside some time to do a regular workout, you'll torch even more calories, and your energy and fitness levels should increase, says Lois Sheldahl, Ph.D., associate professor of medicine at the Medical College of Wisconsin and director of the cardiopulmonary rehabilitation center at the VA Medical Center in Milwaukee. "Fitting exercise into a busy schedule can make such a big difference in the number of calories you burn each day. You'll be able to lose weight faster or just find it easier to maintain your figure," she says.

And remember, exercise offers benefits that go far beyond weight loss—including increased energy, protection against heart disease and diabetes, and a reduced risk of osteoporosis.

The Other Side of Exercise

Unless you're a police officer, construction worker, gym teacher, or carpenter, your normal daily activities won't make a big impact on your cardiovascular health, muscle strength and endurance, or flexibility, which are important for general health, fitness, and disease prevention, says Maggie Greenwood-Robinson, Ph.D., a certified nutrition consultant in Newburgh, Indiana, and author of *Natural Weight Loss Miracles*.

Beating Belly Fat

You do regular aerobic exercise and stomach crunches. You follow a low-fat diet. Yet your belly fat stays. What gives?

Losing fat around your middle depends on your body type and what kind of exercise program you're following. Women are usually shaped like an apple, a pear, or an enviable hourglass. If you have an apple shape, you have a greater tendency to store fat around your tummy. Pear shapes store more fat on their hips and thighs.

Crunches are ideal for strengthening and defining your abdominal muscles, but they won't help banish belly fat. Aerobic exercise burns overall body fat and can whittle your waist. But if the fat still isn't budging, you need resistance training.

Exercise aerobically for at least 30 minutes on most days of the week, and add about 60 minutes of resistance training per week. You can break it up into two or three sessions. Do a series of exercises for your upper and lower body with dumbbells or weight machines. Continue to do stomach crunches. Just add a variety of ab exercises to get the best results.

Expert consulted: Catherine Brumley, certified trainer and fitness director, Canyon Ranch Health Resort in the Berkshires, Lenox, Massachusetts

Aerobic exercise, such as jogging or brisk walking, for 30 minutes or more increases your body's ability to process and utilize oxygen. It keeps your heart and lungs healthy, and it can help prevent diabetes, high blood pressure, and certain types of cancers, says Janet P. Wallace, Ph.D., professor of kinesiology and associate professor and director of adult fitness at Indiana University in Bloomington.

Weight training, on the other hand, is an anaerobic workout because your body doesn't have the same oxygen needs as it does performing an aerobic exercise. Lifting weights builds lean muscle tissue, keeps you strong, gives you more energy, and prevents bone loss—a major concern for women in their postmenopausal years.

Then there are flexibility exercises, such as yoga and stretching, to keep your muscles, ligaments, and tendons limber and less susceptible to injury, says Tia Willows, assistant vice president of group exercise at Bally Total Fitness in Chicago.

Exercise of any type can make you feel really good physically and psychologically after a stressful day. "It allows you to set aside a moment for yourself to relax and unwind. And it's a time to socialize if you participate in an exercise class," says Willows. The effects of exercise may go even deeper than that. Some researchers have shown that it can actually relieve depression and anxiety.

It can also make you look younger. After exercising, your skin tone will take on a youthful glow because working up a sweat increases blood circulation, which supplies nourishment and gives you a healthier appearance, says Dr. Greenwood-Robinson.

How Much Exercise Do I Need?

Increasing the frequency of your workouts, even if you're already active, may help you lose weight. Try to add an hour or two of exercise to your regular routine each week. On average, 2 hours of sustained activity can burn up to 1,000 calories a week. "You must burn 3,500 calories to lose 1 pound of fat. So in 3½ weeks, you can knock off 1 pound through exercise," explains Dr. Greenwood-Robinson.

"Working in up to 2 hours a week of exercise is a very good short-term goal that many people won't find intimidating. If you start by walking or jogging for 20 minutes a day three times a week, you can get fit. You'll become stronger, and you'll be ready to push yourself to do more," says Sherry L. Granader, a nutritionist, certified aerobics instructor, and author of *The Eat Right, Feel Good, Lose Weight, Have Fun Cookbook.*

If you happen to work in a big city and can walk briskly for 10 to 20 minutes to and from your office, you're probably getting all of the aerobic exercise you need. In that

The Math of Weight Loss

If you spend 7 hours a week eating and 1 hour exercising, can you really lose weight? Yes. Weight loss isn't dependent on the time spent eating and exercising. You lose weight by taking in fewer calories and expending more energy with regular exercise.

You could lose a pound a week without exercise by cutting 500 calories a day from your diet. But when you decrease calories too much without increasing physical activity, your body slows its metabolism and stores fat. Exercise turns your body into a more efficient calorie-burning machine.

So eat slightly fewer calories—and get moving. In fact, the more exercise you do, the less you have to worry about calories. By burning 250 to 500 calories a day through excase, set aside 2 to 3 hours a week for weight training and stretching exercises to round out your fitness program, says Willows.

By doing this, you'll condition your muscles and make your body a more efficient fat-burning machine, adds Dr. Wallace.

Now that you know how far a little exercise can go, here are a number of activities experts say you can do to make physical activity fun and exciting. Before starting any exercise plan, however, check with your doctor.

Spinning

You'll be glad to know that twirling around in circles like a top is not the workout we're talking about here. Spinning is an aerobic, high-intensity indoor cycling class. With upbeat music jamming in the background,

ercise, you could lose up to a pound of fat a week—without restricting food.

According to the American College of Sports Medicine, you should get at least 30 minutes of aerobic exercise—such as brisk walking, jogging, or cycling—at least 3 to 5 days a week. If you find it impossible to fit in 30 minutes, break it up. Exercise for 10 minutes at a time in the morning, afternoon, and evening. The bottom line: Physical activity is the best way to burn calories and boost your metabolism to melt away the fat.

Expert consulted: Maggie Greenwood-Robinson, Ph.D., certified nutrition consultant, Newburgh, Indiana, and author of *Natural Weight Loss Miracles*

an instructor takes you through a warmup, hill climbs, descents, intervals of fast and slow riding, and a cooldown at various speeds and resistances. Here's what it does for you.

Health benefits: Spinning conditions your cardiovascular system and tones the muscles in your thighs, calves, buttocks, and hips.

Calorie burn: Spinning burns 260 to 660 calories per hour, depending on your weight and how intensely you pedal.

Convenience factor: Classes are held at various health clubs. If you'd like, you can buy your own stationary bike designed for spinning and work out in the comfort of your own home. But without the direction of a fitness trainer, you may not burn as many calories—or have as much fun. "It's the environment you're in that makes spinning such great exercise. The instructor pushes you, the music pushes you, and the people in the class push you," says Willows.

How often should I do this? Two to three times a week.

Kickboxing

The word may conjure up images of spindly martial arts champions waiting to knock out their opponents or visions of David Carradine demonstrating kung fu in the Old West. But at your local health club or YMCA, kickboxing is a noncontact cardiovascular workout that combines aerobic exercise with shadowboxing to whip you into ringside shape.

It involves a series of kicking, punching, and blocking movements against an imaginary opponent that are choreographed to high-energy music. Classes often go by the names Kwando, Cardio Kickboxing, Cardio Kicks, Boxercise, Tae-Bo, or just kickboxing. Depending on the club, you may wear boxing gloves or hand mitts, use actual punching bags, or combine the movements with step aerobics.

Check out the fitness bonuses you can enjoy by taking a kickboxing class.

Health benefits: Kickboxing is a total-body cardiovascular workout that sculpts and tones your arms, back, hips, thighs, calves, and abs. It also fine-tunes your sense of balance and coordination.

A New Morning Routine Led to Weight-Loss Success

TOPS member Deborah Maier, of Prairie Home, Missouri, struggled with her weight all her life. As an emotional eater since childhood, she often stuffed herself with food whenever she felt scared, stressed, angry, bored, sad, or happy. As a result, she had piled about 370 pounds on her 6-foot frame. And that put her health and her quality of life in jeopardy.

To deal with her weight problem, Deborah took on three challenges: She started eating low-fat, nutritious foods. She dealt with her emotions. And she began a regular exercise program.

In just 18 months, she lost 202 pounds and went from a size 28 to a size 8 dress. Her current weight is 163 pounds. While combining all three strategies helped Deborah lose weight, she believes that it was her daily morning exercise routine that really made the impact.

At 8:00 A.M., Deborah hits the gym, where she runs 3 to 5 miles on the treadmill. After that, she does a series of weight-training exercises and 150 abdominal crunches. By working out in the morning, Deborah believes she has found the key to permanent weight loss.

Calorie burn: You can burn 680 or more calories in a 1-hour class.

Convenience factor: Kickboxing classes are given at various health and fitness clubs across the country. You can also buy or rent kickboxing videotapes and do the routines at home.

How often should I do this? Two to three times a week.

Bowling

Who would have thought that bowling is actually a good workout? Well, repeatedly lifting and hurling a 6- to 14-pound ball, not to mention all that legwork, can do quite a bit for your figure. See for yourself.

Health benefits: You'll tone your throwing arm, hand, and shoulder as you release the ball. You'll strengthen your thighs, butt, and lower back during your approach, knee bend, and finish position.

Calorie burn: Bowling burns 204 calories an hour. Intensity depends on the number of games you play and the number of people you bowl with. More people means longer time lapses between turns, while bowling alone or with just one or two others keeps you moving more consistently.

Convenience factor: You must go to a bowling alley to reap the benefits.

How often should I do this? Two hours twice a week.

Table Tennis

If you have a Ping-Pong table packed away in your basement or garage somewhere, take it out, dust it off, and call a friend. Hitting a small, lightweight ball back and forth across a table actually counts as a real workout. Here's why.

Health benefits: Table tennis strengthens your quadriceps, hamstrings, inner and outer thighs, and hips.

Calorie burn: You can burn 270 calories per hour of steady playing. The type of workout you get is directly related to the level of skill with which you and your partner play. If you really want to start incinerating some calories and improving your game, find a friend who will like to practice a minimum of three times a week for about an hour each time.

Some tables fold up on one side so that you can play by yourself against the upended tabletop. It's a handy option if you can't find someone else to play as regularly as you'd like.

Convenience factor: All you need are a Ping-Pong table, two paddles, some balls, and a place to play.

How often should I do this? Three or four days a week.

Strength Training

Strength training simply means using dumbbells or weight machines or some other form of resistance to strengthen and tone muscles in your upper and lower body. It burns lots of calories, takes years off your appearance, prevents many diseases associated with aging, and is the secret behind many a lean and strong woman, says Dr. Greenwood-Robinson. Here's what it can do for you.

Health benefits: Lifting weights builds muscle. And the more muscle you have, the more calories you burn at rest. It shapes and sculpts your body (don't worry, you won't end up looking like a body builder unless you spend several hours a day in the gym or take steroids), boosts your metabolism around the clock, and helps prevent bone loss. You can shed pounds faster and maintain your weight more easily. And daily activities such as carrying groceries from your car to your front door will never be a problem, says Granader.

Calorie burn: Strength training burns up to 400 calories an hour and builds more muscle tissue. With more body-firming muscle, you're burning more calories, even while doing absolutely nothing.

Convenience factor: You can strength train at the gym or in your own home. All you need are a couple pairs of dumbbells, a weight bench, and a barbell with weight plates. Make sure you have someone spot you when you're using very heavy weights and aren't sure if you'll be able to complete a full set.

How often should I do this? Three 45-minute sessions per week.

Walking

Everyone knows that walking is as simple as putting one foot in front of the other. But if you want to lose weight, you'll have to walk like a woman on a mission—and pump your arms. In other words, power walk. Here's what you can expect if you do it regularly.

Health benefits: Your body will burn more calories and fat throughout the day because of the boost in your metabolism. You'll firm up the muscles in your buttocks, thighs, calves, back, upper arms, shoulders, and abdomen. You'll condition your cardiovascular system, help prevent osteoporosis, elevate your mood, and reduce stress, heart disease, and stroke risk, says Rebecca Gorrell, director of movement therapy at Canyon Ranch Health Resort in Tucson.

Calorie burn: Walking burns 100 calories per mile. You can burn 350 to 450 calories an hour, depending on how fast you walk and on whether you hike on flat or hilly terrain.

Convenience factor: You can walk anytime and anywhere. There's no equipment to buy and no health clubs to join. All you have to do is lace up your walking shoes and head out the door or hop on a treadmill.

How often should I do this? Thirty to 40 minutes four or five times a week. For weight loss, five times a week for 40 minutes a session is recommended, says Gorrell.

Step Aerobics

Choreographed to the beat of heart-pumping music, step aerobics are high-intensity, low-impact exercises that combine dance moves on and around an adjustable platform. The "step" exploded onto the fitness scene in the late 1980s and hasn't lost its popularity yet, says Granader. Here's how this high-energy class can help you drop those pounds.

Health benefits: You'll tone and shape the muscles in your buttocks, hips, thighs, calves, and abs. The arm movements will sculpt your biceps, triceps, and shoulders.

Calorie burn: Depending on the intensity of your workout, you can burn around 600 calories in an hour, using a 6-inch step.

Convenience factor: You can go to the YMCA or health club and participate in a class, or you can buy a step bench and various step videos in some sporting goods stores or catalogs and work out at home.

How often should I do this? Two to 4 days a week.

Jogging

Like walking, jogging is one of the most accessible—and enjoyable—aerobic activities. But that's where the similarities end. Jogging burns calories a lot faster than walking, and it's one of the quickest ways to achieve cardiovascular fitness. Here's how it can pay off for you.

Health benefits: You strengthen and tone your abs and the muscles in your buttocks, hips, thighs, and calves. You build endurance, and your metabolic rate stays super-charged hours after you've completed your workout, says Dr. Greenwood-Robinson.

Calorie burn: Jogging burns 102 calories per mile. Depending on how fast your run, you can burn at least 500 to 600 calories in one hour.

Convenience factor: Jogging is almost as easy to do as walking. There are no lessons to take. No schedules to follow. No complicated moves to learn. Just lace up your running shoes and go.

How often do I need to do this? You can jog 3 to 5 days a week for 20 minutes or more per session.

Your Life Story

Keeping a diary—whether it's a personal journal, a food record, an exercise log, or a combination of all three—really can be a helpful addition to your weight-loss strategy.

"Given that dieting can be a challenge at best and a rather stressful experience at worst, it might be therapeutic to write down your deepest thoughts and feelings about your weight-loss efforts," says Linda Cameron, Ph.D., senior lecturer in psychology at the University of Auckland, New Zealand, who has researched journaling extensively.

Through writing, you can also brainstorm coping strategies for stressful situations. If you're an emotional eater, you can use journaling instead of eating as a way to deal with feelings when you're upset. Finally, writing can serve as a way of monitoring your eating and activities. Keeping a food diary or exercise log can clue you in to bad habits that you might never have realized you had. Then, as you begin to make changes in your lifestyle, you'll see proof of your progress toward a more active, thinner you.

Writing Down to the Bones

Many of us think that we eat less than we actually do. In one study, women miscalculated their daily caloric intake by 620 calories—or more than half an angel food cake.

A food diary can help. Just the act of writing down what you're munching at meals and snacks helps you start making subtle changes in your diet.

If you're ready to raise your consciousness with a food diary, here's what weight-loss experts say you need to do.

Keep Busy with Embroidery

As a military bride living in rural Japan in 1970, Beverly Enos needed a hobby that would occupy lots of time—and cake decorating wasn't what her figure needed. She discovered bunka shishu, a form of Japanese embroidery. Stitched with silk or rayon threads, the wall hangings typically measure 16 by 20 inches or more and resemble delicate paintings. Now 50, Beverly owns her own bunka shishu gallery, Purple Dragon Arts, in Georgetown, Massachusetts, and credits the fine decorative art with helping her permanently lose 70 pounds.

"When I was in Japan, there was very little to do. My husband worked rotating shifts, so I was alone for hours on end. I needed something to do that would take up long spans of time. A neighbor taught me bunka shishu. You can't eat and stitch at the same time!"

You may not live in rural Japan, but you can still use needlework as a weight-loss helper. Try cross-stitch embroidery, needlepoint, crocheting, knitting—anything that keeps your hands busy and your mind off food.

Keep it portable. A 4-inch by 6-inch notebook represents the standard in many studies. You want a diary small enough to carry easily in your purse or pocket, yet with enough space to record everything from your portions to your emotions.

Track essentials. Record the time each time you eat, whether it was a snack or a meal, the food and its preparation method (grilled chicken, steamed vegetables, a chocolate bar), serving size, calories, and grams of fat. A pocket calorie counter can be an invaluable tool to help you keep track of the numbers.

Also include your emotions and exercise. If you jot down how you're feeling every time you eat, you'll soon see if emotions are triggering your snack attacks. Reinforce your new, active lifestyle by scribbling down exercise and activities, noting the calories burned.

Rate your hunger. When you gain, lose, and regain pounds over and over again, it may mean that you're eating on autopilot and have forgotten what hunger feels like, suggests Gloria Kensinger, R.D., a registered dietitian in Wheaton, Illinois. Rating your hunger from 0 to 5 (where 0 equals "starved" and 5 equals "stuffed") can reacquaint you with your body's hunger signals.

Follow food groups. Write your food group goal—for example, "five servings of fruits and vegetables"—in your food diary for every day. Then track your progress: Make a check mark next to your goal each time you choose fruit for dessert or snack on carrots.

Time yourself. You also may want to record how long you spend eating. Perhaps you're nibbling on the run more frequently than you realize or you polish off your food in 15 minutes or less, even when you do sit down to eat. When you learn to eat more leisurely, you'll not only enjoy your food more but also have the opportunity to stop eating when you feel full instead of when it's too late.

Record meals promptly. Jot down the details ("Breakfast: 4 ounces orange juice, a sesame seed bagel with 1 tablespoon cream cheese") immediately after you eat. You'll spend less time on the diary because you won't need to recall what you ate hours ago, and your entries will be more accurate.

Work with a professional. If you're diligent about your food diary, you'll soon have pages of data about your eating habits. But you need more than information to make changes in your lifestyle; you need insight. Here's where a nutritionist can help. After looking at your entries, she can translate your food choices into nutrient intake, food groups, and more so you can see the trends in your own eating patterns and ensure that you're getting the vitamins and minerals you need. "You need some way to evaluate where you are so that you can reach your health and nutrition goals," says Mary Kretsch, R.D., Ph.D., a research nutrition scientist at the USDA Western Human Nutrition Center at the University of California, Davis.

Look for patterns. Do you always eat dinner in front of the TV? Do you reach for chocolate when depressed? Food diaries can help you uncover the situations that can undermine your weight loss. Once you know your high-risk situations, you can develop coping strategies.

Be honest. Fudging your food diary won't make the weight disappear, says Julie Swanson, R.D., a clinical dietitian at Hennepin County Medical Center in Minneapolis. It'll just make it harder for your dietitian to spot problems or offer useful support in your efforts toward a thinner you.

Watch out for burnout. Keeping a food diary will eventually become tiring. Once you've discovered the hidden calories and eating triggers in your life and you've replaced them with healthier habits, you can probably take a break from recording every bite, Dr. Kretsch says. If you hit a weight-loss plateau, though, grab your notebook again; it will help you refocus goals and uncover the source of your weight-loss standstill.

Be kind to yourself. You want your food diary to be accurate, but there's no need to be a perfectionist. "If you tend to be compulsive about eating or counting calories, a food diary can be a negative thing," Swanson cautions. "If keeping a food record is taking away from your goals by making you feel bad, put it away or use it as an occasional spot check to see how you're doing."

Dear Diary

Sometimes, the problem isn't our eating habits but our "feeling" habits.

"Women often eat in a misguided effort to cope with stress," says Simone Ravicz, Ph.D., a licensed clinical psychologist in Pacific Palisades, California, and author of *High on Stress*.

Journaling represents a better way to deal with the stress in your life. Studies have shown that writing about stressful events can boost your immune system, reduce doctor visits, and even lessen the symptoms of chronic diseases such as asthma or rheumatoid arthritis. If journaling can benefit your physical health in such unexpected ways, imagine what it can do for your emotional health and, by extension, your weight loss.

"Writing about the stressful aspects of your life can help you resolve issues and, perhaps in the long run, reduce emotional distress, which is often a trigger for eating 'comfort' foods or overindulging," Dr. Cameron says.

Journaling also provides a way to gain insight and understanding about the issues that you're facing as you lose weight. Perhaps your closest friend has been surprisingly unsupportive of your plans; maybe you're angry at yourself for not shedding pounds faster. Through writing, you can get some perspective on these emotional events. "Putting your feelings and thoughts into words helps you make sense of the experience," Dr. Cameron says. "You're also more able to identify potential coping strategies."

Journaling can be especially beneficial if you suspect that you're an emotional eater. If your food diary shows that you tend to overeat after a fight with your teenager or an outing with your mother, ask yourself why in your personal journal. Once you know the trigger, you can stop the cycle.

If you're ready to start scribbling, here's what journaling experts recommend.

Guilt-Free Pleasure: Romance Novels

Summer or winter, there's nothing more delicious than curling up with a juicy read. Tucked away in a comfy chair, you quickly become engrossed in the latest bestseller—and completely forget about the leftover chocolate cake on the counter.

If you're tired of your usual literary mix, try romance novels. Today's romances feature more diverse characters, plots, and styles than they used to. You'll find heroines who are doctors, lawyers, and single mothers—not just the traditional, simpering servant girls you may remember from your mother's paperbacks.

"Just as women's lives have changed since the 1950s, so, too, have the story lines and characters in romance," says Rosemary Johnson-Kurek, Ph.D., an instructor at the University of Toledo in Ohio and coeditor

Take 20. No time to keep a diary? Think again. Writing for as little time as 20 minutes can improve your mood and health.

Write regularly. If you're dealing with a particularly traumatic experience, you may want to continue writing over a period of 3 to 5 days to allow yourself to work through your different emotions.

Tackle tough topics. To truly benefit from putting pen to paper, you must be willing to write about difficult issues. Rambling about superficial topics simply won't provide the same health advantages.

Be prepared. If you eat in response to stress, carry a notebook with you so that you can write instead of nibble when things get tense. "Writing isn't going to alleviate your hunger pangs, but it may help reduce impulse eating

of *Romantic Conventions.* "Any type of fiction can also be a romance."

Interested in a story with African-American characters? Try Shirley Hailstock or Beverly Jenkins. Have your children gotten you hooked on the *The X Files* with its spooky paranormal plots? Look for Maggie Shayne, whose books feature fantasy elements such as time travel and ghosts. Do you enjoy reading steamy love scenes? Katharine Kincaid is known for her sensual books. Are you a closet fan of the original *Thomas Crown Affair,* with its handsome hero and art theft intrigue? Check out Elizabeth Lowell; her suspenseful adventures often involve jewels and other treasures.

"There's almost anything your heart desires," says Dr. Johnson-Kurek, who enjoys the requisite happy endings. "And there's nothing depressing about them."

triggered by feelings of being unable to cope with stressful situations," Dr. Cameron says.

Don't try to distract yourself. If you're obsessing about food, don't try to divert your mind from food by writing about another topic; it will only make you more likely to run to the refrigerator. Focus on your thoughts and feelings about food instead. Why is it so important for you to eat right now? What does eating mean to you? How can you handle this situation?

Brainstorm solutions. The pessimists among us need a little structure to benefit from journaling. After you write about a problem, keep yourself from lapsing into negativity by spending 5 minutes thinking about new ways to approach the upsetting situation.

Say you're upset at a friend's disparaging comments about your weight. How can you handle this situation now and in the future? After you finish venting in your diary, jot down whatever ideas come to mind. You could take a walk, exercising away your anger rather than drowning it in a bowl of ice cream. Perhaps you could speak to her privately about her unkind words, telling her how hurt you felt and asking her to be more supportive. Maybe you could limit your outings with her—or stop them altogether until she begins acting like the friend you thought she was.

The Art of Snacking

To anyone trying to lose weight, snack foods can seem like little devils luring you toward disaster.

But as often as you say no to temptation, the struggle never gets any easier. "The problem is that snacking is woven into the very fabric of our culture. Many of our social activities center around food, whether it's a coffee break, a sporting event, or a meeting," says Joan Salge Blake, R.D., a registered dietitian and adjunct clinical professor of nutrition at Boston University.

"Women can be very weight conscious, so they feel like they can't eat all those delicious snacks that they see out there. The situation definitely creates a big conflict," says Susan Olson, Ph.D., a clinical psychologist and weight management specialist in Seattle.

So how can you make your life easier in the constant struggle to resist all those beckoning goodies? Easy. Give in.

Make an Angel out of the Snack Devil

Yes, of course eating too many Hershey Bars and Twinkies (or any excess calories, for that matter) between meals can feed into gaining a dress size. But contrary to what many

171

people believe, snacks can actually be healthy and nutritious additions to any weight-loss meal plan.

"The trick is to prepare in advance what snacks you're going to eat. Have yogurt, cut-up vegetables, and chopped fruit on hand so you can dig right in when you're hungry," says Blake.

Second, make your snacks an extension to all your meals. If you plan to eat a bowl of cereal and some fruit for breakfast but can't finish it all, save your fruit for a midmorning snack. If you buy a sandwich, soup, and a salad for lunch, eat your salad a couple of hours later. "It's a strategy that allows you to sneak in the fruits and vegetables that you didn't eat during your meals. And it keeps you from eating the higher-calorie stuff," Blake says.

But if you must have something sinfully sweet, buy chocolate bars and cookies in single-serving packages only. That way, you won't devour a whole box or bag, says Blake. "You'll be shocked to discover how satisfied you are with eating less."

Another snacking bonus: Healthy, planned snacking can prevent you from piling too much food on your plate for lunch and dinner. And that translates into fewer calories consumed.

Tame Those Midnight Temptations

While snacking has many advantages, it also has its disadvantages—especially if you're used to eating rocky road ice cream during late-night talk shows.

Why? Because at night, your body burns far fewer calories than it does during the day, which means that calories from late eating will likely show up on your hips, butt, and thighs, says Audrey Cross, Ph.D., nutrition professor at the Institute of Human Nutrition at Columbia University in

New York City. Here's how you can break the late-night-nibbling habit.

Stop skipping. The biggest mistake you can make is to skip breakfast and lunch. You'll be so hungry at dinnertime that you'll not only eat a large meal but also continue eating for several hours afterward, warns Ashini Shah,

Beat the After-Work Munchies

Why is it that you can you go all day without food at work but turn ravenous the minute you get home? Because you're too busy at work to focus on food. And unless you work around food, it's not nearby to tempt you. Besides, if you really haven't eaten all day, you're starving by the time you walk in the door.

But there's more to the story. Women who skip breakfast and lunch feel deprived and often make mental IOUs to themselves, saying, "I missed two meals. When I get home, I'm going to make up for it."

What's more, when your mind starts to relax, the reality that you're hungry starts to sink in. In fact, all you can do is think about food. So the moment you step foot into the house, you and your appetite are totally out of control. And you risk rushing to the refrigerator and eating everything in sight.

The solution? Eat breakfast and lunch and two healthy snacks to get yourself through the day. Keep apples, bananas, pears, pretzels, or saltine crackers in your car or desk. And before you head home, drink a large glass of water. You'll take the edge off your hunger, and you'll be a lot less likely to raid the fridge.

Expert consulted: Jan McBarron, M.D., director, Georgia Bariatrics, Columbus, Georgia

R.D., a registered dietitian at the Obesity Consultation Center at the New England Medical Center in Boston. And here's the real kicker: Because you'll be making up for lost meals, you'll consume the same number of calories—or more—in one sitting as you would normally eat throughout an entire day, she says.

Another drawback is that missing meals can drastically slow down your metabolism, says Maria Simonson, Ph.D., Sc.D., director of the health, weight, and stress clinic at Johns Hopkins Medical Institutions in Baltimore.

Fill 'er up. If you're not skipping meals but are still raiding the fridge at night, you're probably either eating too little during the day or eating at night for reasons other than hunger, says Blake.

Scrumptious Low-Cal Snacks

Satisfy your sweet tooth or salt craving—and help shrink your waistline—with treats like these.

- ½ cup Häagen-Dazs vanilla raspberry fat-free frozen yogurt: 130 calories, zero gram fat
- ½ cup Häagen-Dazs chocolate sorbet fat-free frozen yogurt: 120 calories, zero gram fat
- ½ cup Edy's coffee fudge sundae fat-free frozen yogurt: 100 calories, zero gram fat
- 1 Weight Watchers Smart Ones Mocha Java Bar: 80 calories, 1.5 grams fat
- 4 oz Jell-O Fat-Free Pudding Snack: 100 calories, zero gram fat
- 1 oz (15 chips) Pringles fat-free potato chips: 70 calories, zero gram fat

The solution? Eat breakfast, lunch, a snack, and then dinner. That way, you won't feel like devouring two bags of potato chips when you're in front of the TV, says Dr. Cross.

Break a sweat. Walk, jog, weight train, or participate in a team sport such as softball, soccer, or volleyball. Physical activity relieves stress and builds self-esteem. As a result, you may be more inclined to eat healthier, says Shah. Accumulating 20 to 30 minutes of exercise daily could help curb appetite and munching.

20 Top Weight-Loss Snacks

The smart way to graze is to choose lower-fat, fiber-rich foods and to eat no more than the recommended serving

38 Snackwell's Zesty Cheese Snack Crackers: 130 calories, 3 grams fat

1 oz (6 chips) Tostitos WOW Restaurant-Style: 90 calories, 1 gram fat*

1 oz (about 18 chips) Guiltless Gourmet Baked Organic Tortilla Chips (red corn, chili lime, blue corn, black bean): 110 calories, 2 grams fat

1 cup popped Orville Redenbacher's 94% Fat-Free Butter Smart Pop: 15 calories, zero gram fat

7 Quaker Crispy Mini Caramel Corn Cakes: 60 calories, zero gram fat

*Contains Olestra, which may cause abdominal cramping and loose stools. Olestra inhibits the absorption of some vitamins and other nutrients.

size, says Kitty Gurkin Rosati, R.D., a licensed dietitian/nutritionist, nutrition director of the Rice Diet Program at Duke University in Durham, North Carolina, and author of *Heal Your Heart*.

Here's how to fit figure-friendly snacks into your weight-loss plan.

1. Freeze your fruit. Arrange grapes on a small cookie sheet and place them in the freezer. Eat them when they're frozen. Store leftovers in a freezer bag for up to 2 months. Serving size: ½ cup grapes; 60 calories, zero gram fat. Another tip: Peel a banana, wrap in plastic, and freeze. Serving size: 1 medium banana; 105 calories, zero gram fat.

2. Roast your veggies. Coat a baking pan with olive oil spray. Arrange chopped or sliced eggplant, bell

Why Do You Wake Up Hungry?

Common sense says it's because you haven't eaten in several hours. But the answer isn't that simple.

Your stomach produces acid after every meal. And the more food you eat, the more acid it makes. If you overate at dinner, the extra acid remains in your tummy all night, along with the normal gastric juices. The end result is stomach acid overload, which can cause strong hunger pangs and a voracious appetite the next morning.

Your hunger also may be caused by fluctuating blood sugar levels. When you overeat, your pancreas pumps out massive amounts of insulin—the hormone responsible for getting glucose into your cells to be used as energy. If your cells reject the glucose (which is common among overweight people), your pancreas dumps out more insulin.

peppers, onions, sweet potatoes, asparagus, mushrooms, and garlic in the pan. Roast at 350°F for 15 minutes, turn them over, and bake for 15 minutes, or until the vegetables are browned. Serving size: ½ cup; 25 to 100 calories, less than 1 gram fat. (Calorie and fat counts will depend on the amount and which vegetables you use.)

3. Savor some cereal bars. The low-fat versions of these fruit-filled snacks come in a wide variety of flavors. Serving size: 1 bar; 130 calories, 3 grams fat.

4. Blaze your own trail mix. Mix three of your favorite low-fat, whole-grain cereals. Look for bran or whole wheat cereals that contain at least 2 to 3 grams of fiber and fewer than 8 grams of sugar per serving. Serving size: 1 cup; approximately 100 calories, 1.5 grams fat.

Meanwhile, excess insulin and glucose are floating around in your bloodstream. Research shows that insulin does two things: It stimulates your appetite, and it produces body fat.

So how do you break this vicious cycle? Drink at least 4 ounces of water and take a chewable antacid, such as Tums, before you hit the sack. This will greatly reduce stomach acid.

To level your blood sugar, eat a breakfast high in protein first thing in the morning. Yogurt, cottage cheese, eggs, and protein drinks made with soy milk are good choices. Don't drink coffee before you eat, or your stomach will churn out that acid again.

Expert consulted: Jan McBarron, M.D., director, Georgia Bariatrics, Columbus, Georgia

5. Scoop some pudding. Try the low-fat and fat-free varieties in single-serving containers. Serving size: 1 container (3.5 ounces); 100 calories, zero gram fat. Also try fat-free instant pudding mix. Serving size: ½ cup; 90 calories, zero gram fat.

6. Pop some corn. Choose the low-calorie, fat-free microwave varieties. Six cups equal fewer than 150 calories. Serving size: 1 cup; 15 calories, zero gram fat. Another option: Air-pop your own popcorn. Then lightly coat the popcorn with olive oil spray and sprinkle it with chili powder, garlic powder, onion powder, pepper, cinnamon, or fat-free Parmesan cheese.

7. Feast on figs. Fat-free fruit bars are available not only in fig but also in cranberry, raspberry, and strawberry flavors. Serving size: 2 cookies; 100 calories, zero gram fat.

8. Grab a bagel. It will fill you up and boost your energy. Serving size: ½ bagel; 105 calories, zero gram fat. Slathering it with 1 tablespoon jelly adds 40 to 50 calories, zero gram fat; 2 tablespoons fat-free cream cheese adds 30 calories, zero gram fat.

9. Jiggle some gelatin. Fat-free and available in myriad flavors. Serving size: ½ cup; 80 calories, zero gram fat. There's also sugar-free. Serving size: ½ cup; 10 calories, zero gram fat.

10. Bake an apple. Core and peel the top third of a large (9 ounces) baking apple. Spoon in 2 tablespoons low-fat granola, 1 tablespoon brown sugar, and a dash of ground cinnamon. Drizzle with 1 tablespoon caramel sundae topping. Cover and microwave for 3 minutes, or until the apple is tender. Serving size: 1 apple; 245 calories, 3 grams fat.

11. Pass the taters. Slice an unpeeled, scrubbed potato into thin wedges and place on a baking sheet spritzed with cooking spray. Sprinkle the wedges with pepper and paprika. Bake at 425°F for 15 minutes, or until tender.

Serving size: 1 potato with spices; about 230 calories, zero gram fat.

12. Make your own chips. Coat a baking sheet with olive oil spray. Cut 24 fat-free, salt-free tortillas into

Planned Snacking Did the Trick

A diet of hamburgers, french fries, fried chicken, and high-fat snacks caused Fran Condo Drozdz, of Litchfield, Arizona, to pile on 30 pounds that she struggled for years to lose. To get rid of her fat, she popped diet pills and tried every fad diet imaginable. The problem was that whenever she lost some weight, she regained it quickly—until she found a more permanent solution: regular exercise, low-fat meals, and lots of planned snacking.

She hasn't looked back since. Fran dropped those 30 pounds 17 years ago, and not one of them has returned. Her 20-year membership with TOPS and her plum position as their health and fitness spokesperson/ambassador has played a key role in her success. She offers women advice on how to keep weight off for good, and she even gives away these weight-loss snacking secrets.

Carry a cooler. Pack a small plastic cooler with you wherever you go, in case you get hungry. Fill it with bagels, jam, apples, bananas, yogurt, and low-fat cheese sticks. You'll avoid stopping at fast-food restaurants, convenience stores, and vending machines.

Prepack your snacks. Select 10 of your favorite low-fat snacks and put 100 calories' worth of each in separate plastic bags. Got the munchies? Just grab a bag and chow down. You'll always know exactly how much you're eating, and you'll never feel deprived. Some of Fran's bagged favorites include pretzels, fig bars, low-fat popcorn, flavored rice cakes, low-fat trail mix, and prunes.

eight pieces each and spread them on the sheet. Bake at 350°F for 10 minutes, or until the chips brown slightly. Remove from the oven, mist with cooking spray, and sprinkle with garlic powder, ground cumin, chili powder, or other seasonings. Serving size: 8 chips; 67 calories, 1 to 2 grams fat.

13. Whip up a dip. Pour into a bowl one 16-ounce can of no-salt, low-fat refried beans and 6 ounces of no-salt salsa. Mix in the juice of 1 lime, 2 tablespoons chopped fresh cilantro, and some minced jalapeño peppers (wear plastic gloves when handling). Serving size: ½ cup; 134 calories, 2 grams fat. Beware of pickled jalapeños; they're loaded with sodium.

Note: No-salt refried beans can be a little difficult to find, but they're definitely worth the effort.

14. Scream for ice cream. Low-fat, low-calorie ice cream, fat-free frozen yogurt, and sorbet are available in decadent flavors. Serving size: ½ cup; 130 calories, zero to 5 grams fat. Frozen yogurt and fruit juice pops, too, are terrific. Serving size: 1 bar; 40 to 100 calories, zero to 1.5 grams fat.

15. Devour some yogurt. Choose low-fat or fat-free varieties. Average serving size: 6 to 8 ounces. Low-fat: 170 to 220 calories, 2 to 3.5 grams fat. Fat-free: 120 calories, zero gram fat.

16. Enjoy some veggies. Buy some precut, bagged fresh vegetables that include broccoli, carrots, and cauliflower. Dip them in your favorite creamy fat-free salad dressing. Serving size (veggies): ½ cup; 35 calories, zero gram fat. Serving size (dressing): 2 tablespoons; 35 to 50 calories, zero gram fat.

17. Munch on rice cakes. Lots of flavors available. Serving size: 5 fat-free mini cakes; 50 calories, zero gram fat.

18. Nosh on nachos. Place 15 baked restaurant-size tortilla chips on a baking sheet lightly coated with nonstick spray. Top each chip with shredded low-fat Cheddar cheese, fat-free bean dip, and salsa. Bake at 325°F for 5 minutes, or until the cheese is melted. Calories and fat will vary with the topping and chips used.

19. Pack pretzels. Available in regular, low-fat, and fat-free varieties. Serving size: 1 ounce; 100 calories, zero gram fat. Dip them in mustard or barbecue sauce.

20. Palm some fruit. Apples, peaches, pears, and oranges are great grab-and-go snacks. Serving size: 1 piece; 100 calories or less, zero to 0.7 gram fat.

Enjoy the Feast

Few things in life are as certain as this fact: You can't escape food during the holidays.

Glossy magazine covers display photographs of the perfect turkey, the ultimate gingerbread house, a Yule log cake. Department stores highlight their gourmet holiday goodies. Tins of baklava, chocolate-covered cherries, and tiny cakes arrive daily at the office. Each weekend brings an open house, a company party, a family celebration.

No wonder we gain a pound a week between Thanksgiving and New Year's. But it doesn't have to be that way. With a little seasonal savvy, we can make our way merrily through the holidays with our weight intact.

Take a Break

While the holidays may bring miracles, you shouldn't expect them weight-wise during the festive season.

"The holidays are problematic for everybody," says Kerri Boutelle, Ph.D., a clinical psychologist at Children's

Hospital in Minneapolis. Seasonal obligations such as shopping or socializing disrupt our normal eating and exercise routines. If we're not traveling to be with family, we're frantically cooking and cleaning for our own holiday fetes. Not surprisingly, weight loss can become more difficult.

That's why many experts advise taking a "maintenance break" during the holidays. Instead of trying to shed pounds in the face of overwhelming temptation, focus on keeping your weight stable from Thanksgiving to New Year's. It sounds simple, but during the holiday season it's a significant accomplishment.

Such a break can benefit your physique and your psyche. Because weight loss often depresses metabolism, a maintenance break "might give your body time to physically adapt to your new body size and allow your metabolic rate to adjust itself," says Josephine Connolly-Schoonen, R.D., clinical assistant professor of family medicine at the State University of New York in Stony Brook. "On the flip side, you'll reduce your own expectations."

By keeping your holiday weight goals realistic, you'll avoid the feelings of failure that often lead to bingeing, and you'll be more likely to stick to your weight-loss plans as your successes build.

More Holiday Helpers

Whether you want to lose 5 pounds or 50, a handful of holiday hints will help you make it to January with your waistline intact. Here's a strategic sampler from weight-loss experts around the country.

Maintain your routine. Don't skip your afternoon walk because you don't have time for your usual 30-

minute loop. Do what you can, even if it's 10 minutes. "Half of what you're doing is preserving the habit of putting on your shoes and getting out the door," says Karen Kemper, Ph.D., associate professor in the department of public health science at Clemson University in South Carolina. "Once you lose a habit, it's hard to reestablish it." Come January 2, you'll have time to resume your regular route, and you'll have maintained the habit.

Keep that diary handy. Even if you don't keep a food journal at any other point during the year, now is the time. In one study, people who religiously used a food diary lost about ¾ pound a week, even during the holidays; the less diligent gained nearly a pound a week.

Bring in reinforcements. As helpful as a food diary can be, jotting down everything you nibble can get tedious. Friendly reminders can keep you motivated. Women and men who received phone calls, comic strips, and postcards from researchers reminding them about the importance of food diaries lost an average of 2 pounds during the holidays, while their counterparts who did not get reminders gained 2 pounds. "Anything you can do to remind yourself to keep your food diary helps, whether it's putting your diary where you can see it every day or leaving reminder notes for yourself around the house," Dr. Boutelle says.

Get ahead of the curve. If you've reached your goal weight, give yourself leeway by losing a few extra pounds prior to the holidays, advises Jan McBarron, M.D., director of Georgia Bariatrics, a medical center for overweight people in Columbus, Georgia, and cohost of the nationally syndicated health talk show *Duke and the Doctor*. "Every fall, I drop 3 pounds before Thanksgiving. Between then and January 2, I can gain that 3

The Truth about Cravings

Does it seem like you crave only things that are bad for you?

Some researchers believe women crave foods such as chocolate because they contain essential nutrients or make women feel good. But others believe sensory, psychological, and behavioral factors are the key—meaning women crave foods that taste good or that are associated with good things like love, holidays, and special memories.

But how do we know that it isn't some chemical in the food that makes us crave it? Researchers at the University of Pennsylvania in Philadelphia gave one group of chocolate cravers a chocolate bar. They gave a second group a capsule containing all the chemicals in a chocolate bar. They gave the third group white chocolate, which has no cocoa (and none of chocolate's chemical compounds). The only thing that relieved the cravings was the chocolate bar. That seems to say that there's something else that's important besides the chemicals.

If a woman allows herself to eat foods that she has labeled as bad, then she feels guilt and shame. Some women are so hypersensitive about "bad" foods that any time they feel like eating such a food, they think they're craving it. All their psychological judgments make them feel that they have a problem, when in fact they don't. So relax a little about your desire to eat foods that you may not feel are the absolute healthiest for you.

Expert consulted: Mindy S. Kurzer, Ph.D., associate professor, food science and nutrition, University of Minnesota, St. Paul

pounds back and be fine. It's not enough to notice, but it's enough to keep me where I need to be," says Dr. McBarron, who lost 70 pounds and has kept it off for more than 10 years.

Puttin' On the Ritz

In December, calendars fill quickly with social occasions: a neighbor's holiday open house, a client's cocktail party,

Why Foods Can Make You Sleepy

With every mix of foods you eat, dozens of chemicals in the brain change. If you feel sleepy, it's usually because you've eaten a fat–carbohydrate combo that's affecting those chemicals.

Starchy carbohydrates, such as bagels, rice, pasta, and potatoes, increase your levels of a brain chemical called serotonin, so you may start to feel sleepy. That's because serotonin is a mood mellower, and there's absolutely no question that it helps you drowse off. The women who eat a carbohydrate-laden lunch are the ones who are in siesta land by 3:00 P.M.

To get more energy from your meals and prevent nap attacks, eat "light" carbohydrates, such as fruits and vegetables. Lean protein sources, such as low-fat string cheese, fish, poultry, and soy products, are also great. The key thing is to avoid high amounts of fat (such as gravy on your turkey) or the combo of high fat and refined sugar in your meals.

Expert consulted: Pamela Peeke, M.D., assistant clinical professor of medicine, University of Maryland, Bethesda, and author of *Fight Fat after Forty*

the company's annual dinner-dance. They're wonderful opportunities to dress up, mingle with friends, and taste a tableful of goodies. What's a holiday gathering without canapés and cocktails?

A chance to escape with my waistline intact, you may be thinking.

Maybe so, but you don't have to forgo the merrymaking because you're losing weight. You simply need to make smart choices about when and how to indulge when you're out and about. Here are some of the smartest choices experts say you can make.

Don't skip meals to "save" calories. You'll arrive at the party ravenous and end up overindulging.

Forget the "new math." It's fine to eat a lighter lunch if you'll be attending an evening event; just don't give yourself too much credit for the calories you banked. "You may have saved a few hundred calories, but you didn't save 1,000," says Connolly-Schoonen. "People often give themselves permission to binge."

Spoil your appetite. A light snack an hour before a party will take the edge off your hunger and help you make better food choices. Try half a sandwich with a glass of fat-free or low-fat milk, a piece of fruit with cheese, or a small bowl of instant oatmeal.

Arrive late. The buffet doesn't look quite so appetizing once the partygoers start picking out the strawberries and spilling sauce on the rice.

Survey the table. By scanning the buffet before you fill your plate, you give yourself the power to craft a healthy, balanced meal that you'll enjoy, instead of worrying about leaving room for the unknown dishes at the table's end.

Go veggie. As always, your best picks will be the raw veggies. They're crunchy, filling, and low-fat—as long as you go easy on the dip.

Be careful of quick breads. Treats such as muffins and pumpkin and banana breads are higher in fat than yeast breads, like wheat and seven-grain.

Think plain. Lean proteins, such as turkey, chicken, and fish—sans the fat-filled creamy sauces and breaded coatings—are healthy choices.

Go nuts. A *small* handful of nuts provides the fat (the healthy kind!) you need to feel satisfied, especially if you're snacking on raw cauliflower and broccoli.

Skirt the buffet. If you're not standing 6 inches from the stuffed mushroom caps and those handy cocktail toothpicks, you won't keep nibbling on them.

Watch the wassail. Drinking alcohol calories (68 in a 3½-ounce glass of white wine) will probably lead you to eat more, according to one study.

Mingle more than you munch. Focus on your friends and colleagues more than the food.

Get romantic. Still can't keep your paws off the buffet? "Hold your date's hand," suggests Melanie Polk, R.D., director of nutrition education at the American Institute for Cancer Research in Washington, D.C.

Facing the Family

As challenging as cocktail parties can be, they're child's play compared with family celebrations. We're not just encountering tempting foods on the table—we're face-to-face with the cooks themselves. "How do you deal with Grandma's pie *and* Grandma, especially when she starts saying, 'Oh, have another slice'?" asks Judith S. Stern, R.D., Sc.D., professor of nutrition and internal medicine at the University of California, Davis. Just the thought of such an exchange makes us quake—and quickly justify the extra calories in the name of family harmony.

A Thinner Thanksgiving Dinner

Jerilyn Tunell, of Independence, Missouri, grew up in a Southern family where lard was the shortening of choice. Those culinary calories added up. By the time Jerilyn was in her thirties, she weighed more than 350 pounds. So she began exploring healthier ways to prepare family favorites. The proof is in the fat-free plum pudding: Jerilyn and her husband have lost 350 pounds between them. Here are her hints on cooking more healthfully this Thanksgiving.

"You almost feel like you can't change family recipes, but you have to get past the emotions. Your grandmother in heaven isn't going to frown if you use low-fat whipped topping on the pumpkin pie, instead of whipped heavy cream! She's going to look down and think you're taking care of yourself."

Jerilyn draws on a host of lower-fat alternatives. She uses applesauce instead of oil in banana bread. She replaces the butter in butterscotch yams with a fat-free butter substitute. She cooks the turkey in Reynolds cooking bags, which keeps the meat moist without basting. Her all-purpose substitute? Chicken broth—it goes into everything from mashed potatoes to gravy.

Although alternatives like leaner meats and butter substitutes can add dollars to the holiday grocery bill, that's okay. "You need to say, 'I'm worth this. My health—my family's health—is worth buying quality ingredients.'"

What did Jerilyn's family think of her first low-fat Thanksgiving feast? "They couldn't tell the difference," she says.

But unless we want to wake up New Year's morning with even more pounds to lose, we need to respond to such scenarios in healthier ways. "You have to chart your course ahead of time," Dr. Stern explains. "You have to be light about it, but you must be determined."

Here's a handful of strategies for sidestepping culinary and familial pressures this holiday season.

Confide in the hostess. Let her know your weight-loss plans. "Tell her that you're watching your weight and to please not be insulted if you don't take large portions," Polk suggests. She'll be less likely to pressure you to eat more than you'd like.

Go potluck. Afraid you'll find nothing you can eat without guilt on your grandmother's groaning table? Provide a side dish that you know is low-cal. "You should be the one bringing the huge bowl of salad," Connolly-Schoonen says. Grandma will appreciate the help, and you'll have at least one healthy option to enjoy.

Compliment the cook. If you're worried about offending your mother by eating less than a plateful of sweet potatoes, take a small portion of food and praise it effusively. "It goes further than eating a huge amount and saying nothing," says Laurel J. Branen, R.D., Ph.D., associate professor of food and nutrition at the University of Idaho in Moscow.

Serve yourself. You can control what and how much goes on your dinner plate.

Taste your favorites. "If this is the only time of year where you get pumpkin pie, you don't want to give that up," Dr. Branen says. Just keep your portion size under control.

Don't clean your plate. If someone gives you more stuffing than you requested, don't finish it out of guilt. Dr.

Branen says that her husband stopped her obsessive clean-plate-club habit with one comment: "He said, 'It can go to waste in the garbage or it can go to "waist" in your body.' He was right. How is that any different?"

Get busy. What Thanksgiving chef could refuse an extra pair of hands after the meal is done? By offering to help with the postfeast cleanup, you'll take your mind off food, and no one will notice that you didn't request seconds of Aunt Edna's fruitcake.

Lie. When all else fails, tell your hostess that you're under the weather. "If you say that you're not feeling well, people understand and don't force extra food on you," Dr. Stern says.

What's Cooking?

If you're the chef this holiday season, you have a wonderful opportunity to make this year's feast a healthier one. Each Thanksgiving, the average American consumes an incredible 4,500 calories and 229 grams of fat—3,000 calories from the meal alone and 1,500 from pre- and post-dinner snacking.

Of course, standing over the stove brings its own temptations.

Dr. Branen recalls one woman who swore that she didn't nibble while she cooked—until she tried wearing a surgical mask while preparing a meal. "You get amnesia when you eat standing up," she says.

If you know you'll be cooking up a storm, experts suggest, try the following to keep your feasting—and tasting—under control.

Distract your tastebuds. You'll be less likely to nibble after you've freshened your breath by brushing your teeth, chewing gum, or sucking on a peppermint candy.

Stop tasting. "You've been making these holiday dishes for years," Connolly-Schoonen says with a laugh. "You probably know how to prepare them by now."

Spice things up. Instead of baking sweet potatoes with butter and marshmallows, try orange or pineapple juice with ginger, mace, and cinnamon.

A No-Cal Holiday Pleasure

When you're trying to lose weight during the holidays, it can seem like every seasonal indulgence, from fruitcake to nuts, is off-limits.

Except for one.

Grandma's pumpkin pie can never compete with the calorie-free treat of kissing your honey under the mistletoe.

With its white berries and golden-green leaves, the plant was helping people celebrate the seasons long before the first Christmas. The Druids, ancient Celtic priests, burned mistletoe at midsummer bonfires. Hundreds of years later, in 18th-century England, young men and women of different social classes used the holiday decoration as an excuse to steal a kiss from someone they could only dream of the rest of the year.

The daring lovers had to act fast. Each bundle of greenery had only so many smooches.

"Each time the mistletoe was used, the couple had to remove a berry," explains Emma L. Powers, a historian with the Colonial Williamsburg Foundation in Virginia. "When the berries were gone, there were no more kisses."

By the way, those berries are poisonous, so if you decide to follow the same tradition, make sure you dispose of them away from the kids and pets.

Choose broth. You'll save fat and calories by substituting low-fat chicken broth for butter when preparing stuffing. Cook mashed potatoes in broth to pump up the flavor, enabling you to skip the butter for mashing.

Bake smart. You can usually reduce sugar in a recipe by one-quarter without affecting the taste, says Stephanie Wilkins, a dietitian in Tuscaloosa, Alabama. She also suggests replacing butter or oil in baked goods with an equivalent amount of applesauce.

Start with soup. You'll feel full faster on fewer calories if you serve a broth-based soup as a first course.

Be inefficient. Dr. Stern clears her Thanksgiving table one dish at a time, making multiple trips between kitchen and dining room to keep her body moving.

Indulge in fresh produce. Fresh out-of-season fruits and vegetables provide a welcome taste of spring or summer in the middle of winter. For a special holiday treat later, you can also freeze your favorite fruit when it reaches its summertime peak.

Lose the leftovers. Each Thanksgiving, Dr. Stern buys new plastic containers, which she promptly fills with leftovers and sends home with her guests.

Establish New Traditions

While treats such as eggnog and pecan pie will always have a place on the holiday table, keeping your new, healthy perspective on eating will be tough if Thanksgiving revolves entirely around the turkey.

Starting new traditions that can help get you off the couch and away from the remote control will help. "Your metabolic rate actually drops below its baseline when you watch TV," Connolly-Schoonen says. "Anything you do is better than turning on the television."

In the spirit of activity, here are some tips for a healthier, happier holiday.

Get active. After the bird's in the oven, take a family walk or start up a game of touch football.

Be creative. Read a story aloud, sing songs, or do crafts as a family.

Volunteer. Many churches and community organizations prepare holiday meals for the homebound or the homeless. Instead of counting calories, you'll be counting your blessings.

Eating Out

Restaurant fare can be a nutritional minefield—typically higher in fat and cholesterol and lower in calcium and fiber than homemade meals. And because Americans typically eat out an average of four times a week, splurging on restaurant meals almost guarantees weigh problems.

"We need to get out of the mindset that every time we eat at a restaurant, it's a special occasion," says Joyce Nelsen, R.D., professor of nutrition and food safety at the Culinary Institute of America in Hyde Park, New York. "Instead, we need to think in terms of what we would eat if we were at home, then put *that* on our plates."

One of the biggest restaurant pitfalls is immense portion sizes. The 16-ounce steak. The ½-pound of pasta smothered with cream sauce. The 8-ounce burger. They're often two to three times larger than dietitians recommend. And we feel we have to finish every last morsel in order to get our money's worth.

"The all-you-can-eat concept is really hurting the American population," says Suzanne Vieira, R.D., director of culinary nutrition at Johnson & Wales University in Providence, Rhode Island. It has contributed to the epidemic of obesity in this country, which in turn is reflected in increasing rates of diabetes and heart disease.

Dining Out on a (Calorie) Budget

That doesn't mean you can never eat out or that you're stuck ordering cottage cheese. "You shouldn't walk away from any meal feeling deprived," Nelsen says, "because that's going to sabotage your weight loss." So have a glass of wine. Split dessert with your date. And most important, take time to enjoy the food and your dining-out experience.

"One of the courses of the meal should be conversation," Vieira says. "Taking it slow prevents what I call unconscious eating, which is when you consume food so fast that your brain doesn't have time to let you know that you're full."

Here's how to deal with huge portions.

Start with soup and a salad. Studies show that foods high in water, such as soup, are more filling, and the fiber in the salad will also make you feel fuller. But make it a clear soup—no heavy cream—and order salad dressing on the side.

Split the entrée. Share your main course with someone at your table—or with yourself the next night. Just have the waiter wrap half before it even gets to the table.

Stick to beginnings. Order an appetizer as your main course. "Most of the time, the appetizer portions are exactly the amount of food you should be eating as an entrée," Nelsen says.

Avoid the potholes. Look out for hidden fat and calories. Go for main courses flavored with salsa, relish, chutney, or sauces derived from natural juices or vegetable reductions. "These flavorings don't have a lot of added fat," says Susan Spicer, a chef at Bayona restaurant in New Orleans. Vegetarian and seafood choices are generally lower in fat, as long as they're not fried. So skip anything that has been dredged in flour or that has breading or batter. "The breading on something like eggplant parmigiana soaks up fat like a sponge," Nelsen says.

The High Cost of Eating Out

Women who eat out at least six times a week take in 300 more calories and 19 more grams of fat a day than women who eat out less often. Plate size is the main culprit. Restaurants' smallest cost is food, so owners beef up entrées to make us think we're getting a better value. A plate of pancakes at a restaurant is more than twice the recommended serving size—that's 370 extra calories before the butter or syrup.

Once all that food is in front of us, our "I've got to get all I've paid for" mentality kicks in. And since we don't have nutrition labels to consult, we don't realize how much damage we're doing to our diets. Who'd think a focaccia club sandwich could have as many as 1,200 calories and 65 grams of fat?

You can avoid overdoing it at restaurants by requesting a nutrition guide from the manager ahead of time. If it's a chain restaurant, you can often check its Web site for nutrition tables or contact the corporation's customer service department. Also, listen closely to your hunger signals. It takes 20 minutes to feel full, so the slower you eat, the less you'll eat. Finally, concentrate more on your dining companions than your food.

Expert consulted: Beth Bussey, R.D., nutritionist, EatRight Program, University of Alabama, Birmingham

Home-Style American

"Plain American cuisine" still ranks as our favorite. But it's loaded with fat and calories and focused on meat rather than healthier whole grains and vegetables. To cut through the fat trap, look for items that are grilled, marinated, or barbecued, says Nelsen.

Best Bets
- Manhattan clam chowder
- Vegetable soup
- Shrimp cocktail
- Hamburger (4 to 6 ounces uncooked weight) with lettuce, tomato, onion, barbecue sauce, and mustard (hold the cheese and mayo)

Battle of the Bulging Restaurant Plates

"Do you make a pasta bowl that holds 80 ounces?" Restaurant-supply companies aren't looking for a family-style serving bowl when they ask that question of the Homer Laughlin China Company in Newell, West Virginia. They're after a single-serving plate, reflecting the trend toward gargantuan servings.

Plates are not only bigger but also deeper, says J. Parry, Laughlin's design director. "Some of the plates are like soup bowls now," he says.

And the standard dinner plate? That's now the *salad* plate at some restaurants.

The reason is that Americans want value—that is, quantity—for their money. So before you go out to eat, practice the words "doggie bag" until you know them by heart.

- Blackened or Cajun chicken with steamed vegetables and baked potato (hold the sour cream)
- Charbroiled pork chops
- Shrimp scampi with rice pilaf

Eating Italian

Italian restaurants are known for their breads, salads, and pastas—all healthy foods in their original states. But you can kiss health goodbye if you smother the bread with butter or olive oil, drown the salad in creamy dressings, or drench a heaping 8-ounce portion of pasta in a creamy Alfredo sauce.

"Pasta may be low in fat, but it still has calories," Nelsen says. Stick with unfilled types, like angel hair, spaghetti, and ziti. Pass up Alfredo, carbonara, and cream sauces in favor of marinara, mushroom, wine, and clam sauces.

Best Bets
- Minestrone
- Shrimp primavera (shrimp and vegetables in a flavored sauce)
- Mussels marinara
- Chicken cacciatore (make sure the chicken isn't breaded)

Chinese Choices

Chinese menus are brimming with healthy choices—if you know where to look. Steer clear of crunchy noodles and anything sweet-and-sour (just another phrase for battered-and-fried). Choose steamed rice or vegetable fried rice over pork fried rice. And check out the menu for lower-fat choices, says Nelsen.

Best Bets
- Egg drop, hot-and-sour, wonton, or Chinese vegetable soup

- Stir-fried chicken and broccoli
- Shrimp or vegetable lo mein (shrimp or vegetables over soft noodles)
- Chicken chow mein
- Vegetarian delight (steamed vegetables with tofu)
- Steamed vegetable dumplings
- One small egg roll with steamed white rice

What French Women Know

These are the secrets that keep French women thin, despite a cuisine famous for cream sauces and rich foods.

Eat at mealtime. No in-between snacking on empty calories.

Choose smaller portions. Even a four-course dinner in France provides only a quarter of the amount of food served in many American restaurants. As for those cream sauces, a French woman would eat about a tablespoon on her chicken; we'd have about ½ cup.

Limit food. No endless bread basket, all-you-can-eat salad bars, or 60-item buffets in France.

End with fruit. Fruit desserts, like pear tarts or poached apples, often replace rich pastries.

Eat slowly. The French are formal about food. Dinner is often a 2- to 3-hour affair—not a sandwich gulped in the car or while watching television.

Drink water. The French are more likely to drink water instead of calorie-packed juice and soda.

Walk. Most French people take public transportation and walk to work, shopping, and entertainment.

Expert consulted: Chris Rosenbloom, R.D., L.D., Ph.D., associate professor of nutrition, Georgia State University, Atlanta

Munching on Mexican

The basic ingredients of Mexican food—corn, chile peppers, and beans—are low in fat and calories, as long as they don't become deep-fried chimichangas or chili con queso, says Nelsen. Skip the nacho chips, go for soft flour or corn tortillas over fried ones, and request black beans instead of lard-loaded refried beans. As for salsa—a tasty compilation of tomatoes, peppers, and onions—eat as much as you want. And don't worry; there are lots of great choices for an entrée.

Best Bets
- Black bean or gazpacho soup
- Chicken, shrimp, or beef fajitas (skip the sour cream and Cheddar cheese)
- Soft taco filled with beans, lettuce, tomatoes, and salsa topped with a sprinkle of cheese
- Chicken enchilada (hold the cheese)
- Arroz con pollo (rice with chicken)
- Bean burrito with a sprinkling of cheese
- Seviche (fish marinated in lime juice)

Food from the Land of the Rising Sun

Japanese food is heavy on vegetables, rice, seaweed, and seafood, and it's light on meat, making it one of the healthiest ethnic cuisines around, says Vieira. Just stay away from tempura, katsu, and agemono. Translation: fried.

Best Bets
- Miso (soy bean soup) or sui mono (clear soup)
- Sushi (rice rolls filled with raw fish or vegetables and wrapped in seaweed paper)
- Sashimi (sliced raw fish served with radish, horse-radish, ginger, or soy sauce)

- Yakitori don (broiled chicken with rice)
- Shakenabe (salmon and vegetables in soybean broth)
- Sunomono (seafood or raw vegetables tossed with a sweet-and-sour vinaigrette)

Tasty Thai

Thai cuisine relies on exotic ingredients like lemongrass and curry to create dishes that are both spicy and sweet. Dishes often feature fruits like mango, papaya, and pineapple, while vegetables, jasmine rice, and seafood also take center stage. Skip anything made with coconut oil or coconut butter, both of which are high in saturated fat, says Vieira.

Best Bets

- Tom yum koong (clear-broth lemongrass soup with shrimp)
- Crystal noodle (chicken noodle with vegetables)

Drink Great Wines instead of Soda

A 3.5-ounce goblet of wine has just 72 calories, compared with 201 in a can of soda. A bonus: The wine will improve not only your dinner but also your health.

Studies show that red wine boosts "good" cholesterol levels and lowers "bad" cholesterol levels, thus reducing your risk of heart disease. That's because wine is chock-full of health-building antioxidants.

Here's how to get the most from wine.

Remember the region. For more antioxidants, choose red wines from Oregon, Ontario, or the Burgundy and Bordeaux regions of France. The cool, damp climates of these areas enable grapes to stay on the vine longer, resulting in increased levels of antioxidants, like resvera-

- Green curry with chicken
- Thai chicken (chicken sautéed with cashews, onions, mushrooms, pineapple, scallions, and chile peppers)
- Garlic shrimp
- Beef basil (sautéed beef flavored with hot basil leaves, fresh hot pepper, mushrooms, and red pepper)
- Vegetable boat (string beans, asparagus, zucchini, onions, and mushrooms in Thai spices)

French Feasting

Cream sauces. Duck legs roasted in their own drippings. Pâté de foie gras. To get around all this fattening fare, look for entrées that are lightly sautéed, and avoid anything with aïoli (a garlic mayonnaise made of eggs and oil), béarnaise sauce (cream sauce made with eggs and butter), or beurre blanc (white sauce that's heavy on the butter), says Vieira.

trol, in the grape skins. If you're unsure about where the grapes for your wine come from, ask a salesclerk or the waiter.

Match your meal. Choose light wines for light food and full-bodied wines for rich food. Pair Beaujolais with grilled vegetables, Riesling with fresh fruit, and white zinfandel with delicate fish like sole, cod, and flounder. Match Chianti with beef stir-fry, Merlot with fatty fish like salmon and tuna, and Chardonnay with vegetable stews.

Maintain moderation. One to three glasses a week is all you need to get the heart-healthy benefits of red wine. Six or more a week, studies suggest, may increase your risk for breast cancer.

Best Bets

- Bouillabaisse (seafood stew)
- Ratatouille (vegetables simmered in olive oil, garlic, and herbs)
- Crudités (marinated vegetables served raw or lightly cooked)
- Rouille (spicy sauce served with fish)
- En papillote (usually fish baked or steamed in parchment paper)
- Coulis (fruit or vegetable puree served over poultry or meat)

Indian Fare

Indian cuisine is big on vegetables, basmati rice, and sauces based on legumes, like chickpeas. Just stay away from korma (cream sauce) and dishes made with coconut. "Coconut oil is the most saturated oil known to man," Nelsen says. Also pass on the pappadam—fried lentil chips—and go with chapati or nan breads, instead of the fried poori or paratha.

Best Bets

- Mulligatawny (lentil, vegetable, and spice soup)
- Dahl rasam (pepper soup with lentils)
- Dahl (a spicy lentil sauce)
- Raita (side dish mixture of yogurt, cucumber, and onion)
- Vegetable biryani or pullao (similar to rice pilaf)
- Tandoori chicken or fish (marinated in spices and slow-roasted in a clay oven)
- Chicken or shrimp saag (spinach)
- Saag panir (a spinach dish featuring cheese made with milk and lemon juice)
- Chicken or fish masala (a red sauce generally lower in fat)

Save Room for Dessert

Indulging in dessert won't blow your diet, as long as you make smart choices. If you must have that chocolate torte, split it with someone or have it only on very special occasions, suggests Susan Lifrieri-Lowry, chef coordinator and pastry chef at the French Culinary Institute in New York City. Even better, satisfy your sweet tooth with one of these delectable, relatively low-fat and low-calorie desserts.

Best Bets

- Vacherin (a meringue shell filled with fruit or sorbet)
- Fruit tart
- Fruit crisp
- Baked apple
- Poached pear
- Fruit soufflé
- Roasted fruit or compote in a phyllo shell
- Crème caramel or flan (rather than crème brûlée)
- Sorbet

New Research in Medicine

To any woman who has wrestled with the scale, a prescription for a weight-loss drug that can quickly melt pounds away sounds like a miracle. No more "dieter's platters" of cottage cheese and peach halves. No more sweaty 5:00 P.M. aerobics classes. And all the chocolate ice cream we can eat. Sounds too good to be true!

Which, of course, it is.

"The reality is that anyone who takes medication to lose weight will end up doing the same things that anyone else does to lose weight: namely, altering their eating habits and exercising, once the medications are discontinued. That's the part most people don't realize," says Evelyn L. Lewis, M.D., university health center director at the Uniformed Services University of the Health Sciences in Bethesda, Maryland, and a weight-loss researcher. "When the medications are discontinued, the majority of patients tend to regain the weight they've lost—and more—because they haven't adapted to a change in their lifestyle behaviors."

New Thinking, New Treatments

In the past, physicians were reluctant to prescribe drugs for weight loss. "People used to think that losing weight was a matter of willpower," explains Caroline M. Apovian, M.D., director of the Nutrition and Weight Management Center at Boston Medical Center and associate professor of medicine at Boston University School of Medicine. "Many doctors felt the same way."

But physicians and researchers are beginning to revise their thinking.

Discoveries of hormones and proteins that influence everything from appetite to metabolism have opened new worlds in obesity research and potential treatments. At the same time, despite a never-ending parade of diets, Americans are in the middle of an obesity epidemic.

Dr. Apovian believes that it is vital to the control of this epidemic. He suggests medical professionals treat obesity as a chronic disease, like diabetes or high blood pressure, instead of writing it off as a symptom of weak willpower.

"What's so different about taking drugs for obesity?" Dr. Apovian asks. "People with hypertension take drugs. People with diabetes take drugs. Why is it that obese people can't take drugs to manage their disease?"

Although the first generation of weight-loss drugs comprised mostly amphetamines, which can be highly habit-forming, the current generation tends to be much safer. "When the amphetamines came out, no one really understood their truly addictive nature," says Denise Bruner, M.D., president of the American Society of Bariatric Physicians and a physician practicing in Arlington, Virginia. Now if your doctor prescribes medication to help you lose weight, she'll probably give you one of three options: orlistat, a fat blocker; sibutramine (Meridia), which helps you feel full faster; or phentermine (Phentride), an appetite suppressant.

Should You or Shouldn't You?

The decision to take weight-loss drugs depends on multiple factors. Your dieting history is important, but so are your weight, your health, and, most important, your willingness to change your lifestyle.

Still, they're drugs, which means that they carry risks as well as benefits. Before you take a single pill, your doctor will want to give you a thorough medical screening, checking for everything from heart problems to high cholesterol. She'll also calculate your body mass index (BMI) and ask about your health. Doctors generally reserve weight-loss drugs for those who are severely overweight (a BMI of 30 if you're otherwise healthy or 27 if

Medicines That Make You Fat

It's just not fair. Certain classes of drugs can lead to weight gain.

Some medications can affect your appetite or the feelings of fullness that tell you when to stop eating. The older tricyclic antidepressants, for example, may lead to an increased appetite. So can lithium, typically prescribed for depression or bipolar disorder, and antipsychotic drugs such as clozapine, often prescribed for schizophrenia.

Other drugs affect how fat is stored or distributed in your body. Corticosteroids (typically prescribed for rheumatoid arthritis, allergies, or asthma) increase your appetite and shift where your body stores fat. Your body moves fat to your torso, putting you at greater risk for cardiovascular disease. And these medications put you at greater risk for diabetes.

you have conditions, such as diabetes or high blood pressure, that can be helped by losing weight). So, if you're just trying to lose 10 pounds, forget antiobesity meds; it's back to the treadmill for you.

Even if you meet the BMI requirements, you can't turn the treadmill into a plant holder or fill the freezer with full-fat ice cream. Your doctor may be writing the prescription, but she'll expect you to be an active participant in your weight-loss efforts. The drugs may give you a jump start on your weight loss, but you need to adopt a healthier lifestyle that will work in concert with your medication, says Mary Wangsness, M.D., a bariatric physician in St. Paul, Minnesota.

If you have diabetes, you would expect to gain weight when you get your blood sugar under control with medications. With uncontrolled diabetes, calories go out in the urine. Once your insulin level is stabilized, you start storing the calories that your body had been wasting. Wait until you get your diabetes under control before you address stabilizing your weight.

If you're considering a hormonal contraceptive such as Depo-Provera, be aware that many women gain 5 to 10 pounds in their first year on this birth control method.

Talk to your doctor about alternatives if you think your prescription is making you gain weight. Eating less and exercising more will help, too.

Expert consulted: Julie Oki, Pharm.D., associate professor of medicine, University of Missouri–Kansas City School of Medicine

What's Wrong with Fen-Phen?

To many dieters, the drug combo fen-phen was a dream come true. Thanks to the appetite suppressant phentermine (phen), they simply didn't feel hungry. When they did eat, fenfluramine (fen), with its serotonin-boosting effects, helped them feel full sooner.

"My patients on fen-phen didn't care about food. Many had to force themselves to eat," remembers Mary Wangsness, M.D., a bariatric physician in St. Paul, Minnesota.

But fen-phen, which was never approved by the FDA for combination therapy, had serious consequences. In 1997, researchers found that some fen-phen users had leaky heart valves. As a result, drug manufacturers pulled fenfluramine and a related drug, dexfenfluramine, from the market. Phentermine, which is considered safe when used alone, remains in use.

Other fen-phen users developed high blood pressure in the blood vessels of the lungs, which makes it hard for the

Orlistat: Stop Fat Before It Starts

"A moment on the lips, a lifetime on the hips," the old saying goes. Unless, that is, you're taking orlistat, one of the newest kids on the weight-loss block.

What it does: A weight-loss drug known as a lipase inhibitor, orlistat prevents your body from absorbing as much as 30 percent of the fat in the foods you eat. In one study, men and women on the drug lost an average of nearly 20 pounds in the first year of treatment. It sounds like the ultimate wonder drug—until the "gastrointestinal events" begin.

What to expect: "If you eat a Big Mac while you're taking orlistat, you're in for a big shock," Dr. Wangsness

heart and lungs to provide the oxygenated blood we need to live.

There is some good news: Preliminary evidence from studies suggests that heart valves damaged by the drug combo may heal themselves, says Christina Wee, M.D., instructor of medicine at Harvard Medical School—although she emphasizes that the jury is still out on this matter.

"With fen-phen, by the time you realize you have valvular heart disease, it may already be severe," says Dr. Wee. If you used fen-phen, talk to your doctor. She may want to screen you for valve problems, especially if you used the drug for longer than 6 months or expect to have dental work or surgery in the near future. As a precaution, ask about preventive antibiotics before any invasive procedure. Otherwise, bacteria that enter your bloodstream may become lodged in a damaged valve that you didn't know you had.

says. Your body is absorbing only 70 percent of that fat, and the other 30 percent has to go somewhere. Which leads to the most common side effects: oily or fatty stools, oily spotting, and increased urgency in bowel movements.

Make it work for you: If you're eating responsibly and sticking to a diet with 30 percent fat or less, you don't need to worry about "orlistat's revenge." "Most people are afraid of the side effects, so they watch their diets," Dr. Wangsness says. As a result, you develop better eating habits, lose weight, and often improve your cholesterol levels and blood pressure.

One more thing: When orlistat eliminates that 30 percent of the fat, you also lose valuable fat-soluble vitamins, such as A, D, E, and K. It's recommended that you take a multivitamin whenever you are on a weight-loss program.

Sibutramine: Feel Full Faster

Perhaps potato chips and other high-fat foods don't fill you up. Then again, neither does anything else. No matter how much you eat, you never seem to feel full.

You might want to talk to your doctor about sibutramine (Meridia).

Leptin: Big Promises, Little Reality

When researchers discovered leptin in 1995, they thought they had solved the obesity equation. Leptin, a hormone found in fat cells, seemed to influence both appetite and metabolism, leading to weight loss in obese mice injected with the substance. Researchers hoped it could do the same for people.

"Leptin is probably the greatest discovery in obesity, but it's probably not going to help women lose weight," says Eleftheria Maratos-Flier, M.D., associate professor of medicine at Harvard Medical School and an investigator at the Joslin Diabetes Center in Boston.

Instead of controlling appetite or metabolism directly, leptin primarily tells your brain how much energy—or fat stores—your body has. Then your brain decides whether you have enough body fat to perform the "extras" of life, such as menstruation or carrying a baby. So the amount of leptin in our blood generally corresponds to our percentage of body fat. If we're thin, we have little leptin; if we're heavy, we have lots.

What it does: Sibutramine prevents the intake of serotonin and norepinephrine—mood-lifting hormones—into your appetite center, thereby increasing your feeling of fullness. It also increases your heart rate and blood pressure, making this drug a poor choice for someone with heart problems or uncontrolled high blood pressure.

What to expect: You'll still feel hungry, but thanks to increased levels of circulating serotonin and norepinephrine, you'll feel full faster and, hopefully, eat less. You won't lose dramatic amounts of weight; in one study, people lost an average of 10 to 14 pounds in a year, depending on how much sibutramine they took.

But if we're born without any leptin (a rare genetic disorder), the brain thinks we're starving and tries to save us. Metabolism slows down, and we eat uncontrollably. Give us leptin and the pounds drop off as we start eating and burning calories normally.

Unfortunately, if you give leptin to a normal overweight person, you won't see such dramatic effects. Men and women who received the highest doses of leptin in one major study lost an average of only 15½ pounds in 6 months—less than a pound a week. "Leptin hasn't worked well as a therapy because most people have pretty high leptin levels," Dr. Maratos-Flier explains. "Giving them more doesn't do anything."

Leptin may eventually prove more effective in preventing weight regain in people who have dieted, Dr. Maratos-Flier suggests. Raising leptin levels in a woman's blood could trick her brain into thinking that she hasn't lost the weight.

Make it work for you: Although sibutramine is considered an appetite suppressant, you'll still get hungry; you just won't need to eat so much to feel sated.

One more thing: If you're currently taking any drugs for depression, it's necessary to check with your physician before taking sibutramine.

Phentermine: Reduce Your Hunger Pangs

Phentermine grabbed headlines in 1997 as the second syllable of the popular diet drug combo fen-phen when fenfluramine—the "fen" part—was recalled.

Used independently, phentermine remains a safe and effective weight-loss drug for short-term use.

What it does: Considered a "second generation" obesity drug, phentermine chemically resembles the amphetamines that doctors initially prescribed for weight loss. It raises your blood pressure, increases your heart rate, and suppresses your appetite.

What to expect: What if you simply didn't feel hungry? For women who feel deprived when they diet, ravenous as opposed to hungry, and unable to control their appetite, phentermine can help.

Make it work for you: The effects of phentermine, like those of many weight-loss drugs, seem to plateau at around 6 months, so if you haven't been exercising and eating right, you will probably experience problems keeping the weight off.

One more thing: If you're a former fen-phen patient who wants to try antiobesity medications again, you might consider phentermine.

The Next Generation?

If you've tried all three of these medications with no success, don't throw up your hands in despair. Obesity researchers are constantly discovering more about the intricate relationship between the brain and weight. Soon they may be able to create a new generation of weight-loss treatments that target specific mechanisms in the brain that lead to obesity.

One of those mechanisms is leptin, a hormone that tells your brain how much body fat you have, allowing the brain to regulate how much you eat and how many calories you can burn.

"We didn't even know it existed until recently," says Sheila Collins, Ph.D., associate professor at Duke University Medical Center in Durham, North Carolina. Now researchers just have to figure out how to successfully manipulate the complex hormone.

It may be a while before any new discovery leads to a safer and more effective obesity treatment, however. Weight gain is a very complex process, and we just don't yet know how all the pieces of the puzzle fit together.

The bottom line? Don't postpone your weight-loss plans to wait for the next miracle drug. Regardless of what weight-loss drug our doctors may prescribe for us in the future, Dr. Collins says, "there will always be a place for diet and exercise."

Supplements

Intellectually, we know the kind of lifestyle changes we need to make to lose weight: Move more and eat fewer calories. But in our hearts, we lust after the easy solution.

Manufacturers understand our longing. That's why dozens of dietary supplements crowd store shelves, enticing us with promises to sate hunger, speed metabolism, and absorb fat before it has a chance to find our thighs and butt.

While old friends, like meal-replacement drinks and heart-racing drugstore pills, are still out there, the hottest area in weight loss today is in so-called natural supplements containing ingredients like ephedra, chromium picolinate, hydroxycitric acid, and chitosan.

"Natural supplements are presumed to be safe because they come from nature in their original form," says Laurie Fan, director of content management at BioValidity.com and publisher of the *BioNutritional Encyclopedia* and other life science databases on the Internet.

And some *are* safe, says Gail Mahady, Ph.D., assistant professor of pharmacognosy at the University of Illinois at

Chicago. "But some of the most potent toxins come from plants."

Not to mention that most of these supplements don't work as manufacturers promise they will.

Ephedra

Of all the "natural" weight-loss substances, the herb ephedra is the most controversial. Commonly known by its Chinese name, *ma huang*, it has been used in China for more than 5,000 years to treat bronchial asthma and other upper respiratory conditions. But, ironically, never for weight loss.

Yet in this country it's found in hundreds of diet supplements, powders, drinks, and diet bars along with other stimulants that claim to decrease appetite, raise metabolism, and burn fat.

Its active ingredient, ephedrine, stimulates the cardiovascular and central nervous systems, which may speed heart rate, boost blood pressure, and induce nervousness, insomnia, headaches, or dizziness. In high doses it may contribute to stroke, heart attack, seizures, and even death, says Dr. Mahady.

And its effects on weight loss are disappointing.

That's why some manufacturers combine it with caffeine and aspirin to make thermogenic supplements called E-C-A, which raise metabolism and burn fat. In fact, ephedrine and caffeine do work together to increase metabolism and decrease appetite, says Carla Wolper, R.D., a nutritionist at the Obesity Research Center at St. Luke's–Roosevelt Hospital Center in New York City. She cautions, however, that adding aspirin to the mix can cause stomach problems in some people. And because both caffeine and ephedra are stimulants, you eventually build up a tolerance to them.

Another problem: Like many ephedra-based supplements, the mixture may cause irregular heartbeat, anxiety, and jitteriness. Since 1994, the FDA has received more than 800 complaints from people experiencing side effects from taking ephedra-based products.

Talk to your doctor before taking any over-the-counter weight-loss aid. And since ephedra can create so many serious health problems, you should use it only under the guidance of a qualified practitioner.

Chromium Picolinate

Several studies suggest that this supplement, a form of the mineral chromium, builds muscle and reduces fat. Chromium assists in deriving energy from carbohydrates

Don't Overeat

You're more likely to overeat if you eat too fast, skip meals, or wait too long between meals. Wolfing down food doesn't leave enough time for your brain to signal your stomach you're full. This communication usually takes about 20 minutes.

Skipping meals or waiting too long between meals means you're ravenous when you hit the table. By the time that signal saying "enough" hits your brain, you've even eaten tomorrow's leftovers.

Here's how to break the cycle.

Eat regularly. If you might miss a meal, carry with you some healthy snacks like peanut butter and apples or low-fat yogurt. Make sure that your snacks include protein—it keeps you full longer than carbohydrates alone.

and fats, improving your body's response to insulin so that your blood sugar level remains steady.

Weight-loss studies are mixed, however. Some researchers think that this supplement works only if your diet is already chromium deficient. Others say that it depends on the type of chromium used, dosage, and length of time it's taken. Still others conclude that it just doesn't work as well as the mainstays of weight loss: exercise and a low-fat, high-fiber diet.

Yet they do agree on one thing: It's safe.

Recommended dose: 400 to 600 micrograms per day. Don't expect immediate results; you'll need to take it for nearly 6 months before you see a change, says Richard A. Anderson, Ph.D., lead scientist at the USDA Human Nutrition Research Center in Beltsville, Maryland. Doses above 200 micrograms should be taken with medical supervision.

Eat between meals. Try those same snacks even if you don't miss a meal. Eating something every 3 to 4 hours keeps your blood sugar stabilized and prevents overeating at the next meal.

Slow down. Chew your food slowly. Talk to people or put your knife and fork down between bites. Get up and walk around the house twice before you reach for seconds.

Get out of the kitchen. Take your plate to another room. Suddenly, getting seconds might be too much of an effort.

Expert consulted: Michele L. Trankina, Ph.D., nutritional consultant and professor of biological sciences, St. Mary's University, San Antonio

Chitosan

This fiberlike substance comes from the shells of lobster, crab, shrimp, and insects. It supposedly helps you lose weight by absorbing fat in your digestive tract.

Sounds good in theory. But here's the problem: Chitosan binds not only fat but also essential vitamins that need fat to get into your cells. We're talking about vitamins such as A, D, E, and K, as well as important phytonutrients like carotenoids that protect against cancer and other chronic diseases, says Michele Trankina, Ph.D., nutritional consultant and professor of biological sciences at St. Mary's University of San Antonio.

"People may be tempted to take more of these vitamins to make up for what they lose through the chitosan," Dr. Trankina says. Don't. "Some fat-soluble vitamins can be toxic—and even fatal—taken in high doses."

And it's not even certain that chitosan really helps with weight loss. Of three European studies examining chitosan's effects, only one found any benefit. And in that case, it's possible the biggest contributor to weight loss was the very low calorie diet the people followed. When researchers tried a similar study without restricting calories, no one lost any weight.

Pyruvate

Pyruvate is a natural substance resulting from the breakdown of carbohydrates in your body. It's found in the blood, heart, brain, and liver. It's even found in foods, such as red apples, red wine, Cheddar and provolone cheeses, bananas, and garlic.

To date, research has shown that pyruvate is a safe and effective weight-loss supplement when combined with a healthy diet and regular exercise. It's a natural metabolism booster, and it prevents your body from producing fat, says

Judith E. Arch, R.D., a bionutritionist at the University of Pittsburgh General Clinical Research Center.

In one study, overweight women who took pyruvate lost 37 percent more weight and 48 percent more body fat than those taking a placebo. The supplement seems to help even without a low-calorie diet, says Ronald Stanko, M.D., associate professor at the University of Pittsburgh Medical Center and principle author of pyruvate studies.

Another pyruvate benefit is that it preserves muscle mass—your own fat-burning system—which many women

Who Regulates the Diet Supplement Industry?

Uh, no one. In 1994, Congress passed the Dietary Supplement Health and Education Act (DSHEA), putting supplements like ephedra and pyruvate in the same category as food. Thus, although they fall under the jurisdiction of the FDA, manufacturers can market their products without prior approval from the FDA, without any premarketing testing, and without even proving that the product is safe.

There's also no manufacturing oversight, as there is with prescription drugs, to ensure quality. So no one is actually checking that an herb's active ingredient was used in the preparation or that a pill actually contains the dosage described on the bottle.

"Right now, people are on their own. And some of the worst offenders are in the weight-loss industry because there's such demand. People still want the magic bullet," says Ruth Kava, R.D., Ph.D., director of nutrition for the American Council on Science and Health in New York City.

lose when they rely on low-calorie, no-exercise programs for weight loss, Dr. Stanko says.

Sounds almost too good to be true—and it may be.

"You can't just rely on the pill," Arch says. "You really have to eat a healthy diet rich in fruits, vegetables, and whole grains. And you should keep your activity level up. Otherwise, you'll be disappointed."

Recommended dose: 4 to 6 grams a day, according to Dr. Stanko.

Guarana

Nicknamed "zoom" because of its tendency to perk you up faster than a triple espresso, guarana is a dried paste made from the crushed seeds of *Paullinia cupana*, a woody shrub native to Brazil and Uruguay.

It gets its name from the Guaranis South American Indians, who have used it for thousands of years as an aphrodisiac, diarrhea treatment, and sustenance during long fasts.

Today you're most likely to find it in South American carbonated drinks, where its high caffeine content provides a quick jolt. In this country, however, we've grabbed on to it for weight loss.

There really aren't any published studies showing that guarana works for weight loss.

Its use is associated with possible side effects like anxiety, nervousness, insomnia, stomach upset, headaches, and heart palpitations. It's often sold in combination with ephedra and other stimulants, which usually worsen these symptoms and may cause other health problems. Long-term use of excessive amounts isn't recommended because guarana's caffeine stimulates the nervous system. Guarana can also irritate the gastrointestinal tract. Avoid guarana if you have heart disease or if you're sensitive to caffeine or are pregnant or nursing.

Hydroxycitric Acid

Called HCA for short, most hydroxycitric acid comes from the tropical fruit *Garcinia cambogia*, commonly known as the brindall berry. It's a modified form of citric acid, which turns the food you eat into the calories you burn or store as fat.

Basically, by blocking a certain enzyme that normally converts citric acid to fat, HCA prevents your body from making fat. Animal studies support these claims, but the substance hasn't lived up to its promise in humans.

"There's really no evidence proving that HCA actually works," Dr. Mahady says. "So at this point, I wouldn't recommend buying it."

Meal-Replacement Drinks

Ah, if only we didn't have to prepare, cook, and clean up meals. Enter meal-replacement drinks like Ultra Slim Fast and Nestlé Sweet Success.

The good news: They're enormous time-savers, they don't contain any harmful drugs or herbs, and they come in a variety of flavors, including chocolate.

The bad news: They might not make you feel any less hungry.

Chock-full of vitamins and minerals, yet low in fat, they're touted as substitutes for breakfast and lunch. And it's true; if you occasionally substitute a 200-calorie drink for a 1,000-calorie pastrami sandwich, you will eventually lose weight. But Wolper is concerned that the regular use of diet drinks causes you to miss the benefits of eating a wide range of food.

"I don't recommend any woman stay on this plan for any length of time," Wolper says. "You'll miss out on a wide variety of foods that contain important nutrients."

PART FOUR

The Beat Goes On

The Cycles in a
Woman's Life

When many of us hit our forties, all the birthday presents and cards in the world can't disguise one significant fact: We've gained weight. No longer can we get away with eating that extra slice of pepperoni pizza on Monday, that double cheeseburger and large fries on Friday, or that chocolate ice cream sundae on Saturday.

In our twenties, however, we could eat! Late-night parties where the four food groups were nachos, potato chips, sour cream dip, and beer. Decadent Sunday brunches of chocolate chip pancakes with a side of bacon. Then we'd slip into another size 4 pair of jeans and head out for a day of antiquing or hiking or any of the other thousand things we used to do before we had kids and soccer games and husbands and houses and dogs to fill our weekends. If we gained a few pounds, no problem. A couple of nights at the gym, a jog along the beach, and—poof!—the extra weight was gone.

No more. Now, in addition to the fullness of our lives, we've added the fullness of our figures, mainly around our hips, butts, thighs, and pouchy stomachs.

Even more discouraging: Those pounds seem like they're stuck to us with superglue. Why?

We Just Don't Move the Same Way

For starters, we're not as physically active as we were in our early twenties. Then, we were likely to go jogging, walking, cycling, and swimming with friends. Now we're lucky if we get out of the car or move away from the computer because we're so focused on our careers and families, says Pamela Peeke, M.D., assistant clinical professor of medicine at the University of Maryland in Bethesda and author of *Fight Fat after Forty*.

"Many women are working and sitting on their bottoms all day long," says Dr. Peeke. "The lawyer becomes a judge, so she's no longer standing in court. And when she goes out, it's for a lunch meeting, not a night out on the town."

Then there are our kids. Pregnancy often pads our bellies, hips, and thighs with fat that only daily exercise will budge. In fact, it brings one of our worst nightmares to life: It creates new fat cells that may *never* die. That's one reason it often takes 10 years to lose the weight that we gained in 9 months.

And, of course, there's perimenopause, that 5- to 10-year period before menopause actually hits. During this time, our hormones are fluctuating as wildly as when we were teenagers. Only this time, instead of speeding things up, they're slowing things down—specifically metabolism, the rate at which we burn calories.

"Starting at age 20, a woman's basal metabolic rate declines 5 percent per decade," says Dr. Peeke. "Sedentary women can experience as much as a 10 percent decrease. And that's purely age-related." The slower your metabolism, the harder it is to burn those calories.

Cheer up. There are many positive steps that we can take to slow down the normal aging process and meet our weight-loss goals. They just require a little more of that wisdom and ingenuity that we've amassed with age.

Curling Iron

Muscle should be considered a hot commodity because it incinerates calories. Every pound of muscle on your body burns at least 35 calories a day; a pound of fat burns about 2. And that's just while you're lying on your back, reading the latest *Cosmo*.

Fat Can Be a Good Thing

Carrying around a few extra pounds in your menopausal years can be an advantage. If you're physically active, no more than 20 pounds overweight, and your additional padding is on your hips and thighs instead of your abdomen, you'll have more estrogen in your body than your thinner counterparts. Estrogen resides in fat, which may mean fewer hot flashes, less vaginal dryness, and a lower risk for developing osteoporosis, says Denise Bruner, M.D., president of the American Society of Bariatric Physicians and a physician practicing in Arlington, Virginia.

Body fat also offers some protection against osteoporosis by acting as a reserve bank when you don't meet your nutritional needs. There are certain times when your muscles pull what they need from your fat stores, instead of your bones, to sustain themselves, which keeps your bones intact, says Dr. Bruner.

What's more, added fat preserves vitamin D, needed for calcium absorption.

That's one reason we could eat whatever we wanted when we were younger and still not gain weight, says Denise Bruner, M.D., president of the American Society of Bariatric Physicians and a physician practicing in Arlington, Virginia.

But beginning around age 20, thanks to a combination of aging and sedentary lifestyle, we start losing lean muscle—about 5 pounds every decade. By the time we hit our forties, we're burning 350 fewer calories a day than we did in our twenties. By our sixties, we'll be burning 700 fewer calories. This adds up to 36 more pounds of weight every decade if we don't change our eating and exercise habits.

"You go from being a metabolic furnace in your twenties to a glacier in your forties and fifties," says Dr. Peeke.

The good news is that you can regain every pound of muscle that you've ever lost, and then some, through

Lose Just 10 Pounds

If your doctor says that you must lose weight for your health, don't press the panic button. All you probably need to do is drop 10 pounds. That's all it takes to lower your blood pressure, cholesterol, and blood sugar levels, says Pamela Peeke, M.D., assistant clinical professor of medicine at the University of Maryland in Bethesda and author of *Fight Fat after Forty*.

What's more, the first 10 pounds lost will help you place less stress on your hips and knees and thus help prevent painful osteoarthritis. You'll gain more energy, boost your self-esteem, and decrease your risk of heart disease, stroke, and cancers of the breast, ovaries, endometrium, and colon.

weight training. Devoting just 20 minutes three days a week to strengthening your arms, shoulders, back, stomach, chest, and legs can help you build about 1 pound of muscle every month. After 2 months, your body will burn 70 calories more a day.

If you add aerobic exercise—like brisk walking, jogging, or cycling—to your weight routine, you'll burn up to an additional 300 calories per 45-minute session. "It will keep you metabolically hot," says Dr. Peeke. "You want your muscles rocking and rolling."

The Hormonal Roller Coaster

At some point in our forties, that delicate balance of female hormones goes awry. Estrogen levels start to drop, along with progesterone, DHEA (dehydroepiandrosterone), and thyroid and growth hormones, all of which can dramatically slam the brakes on your metabolism. Here's how each affects your weight.

Estrogen. Falling estrogen levels can rearrange body fat. The fat that once graced your hips and thighs in your twenties and thirties suddenly makes a beeline for your stomach, changing your pear shape into an apple. Why? The less estrogen you have, the more certain enzymes make your stomach area suck up the fat.

Too much fat around tummies is toxic, says Dr. Peeke, because it can set us up for heart disease, diabetes, and cancer later in life. "So women have to be on the red alert to keep that fat down to a minimum."

Thyroid hormone. Your thyroid gland, a butterfly-shaped organ nestled at the base of your throat, is a metabolism regulator. When all goes well, the gland pumps out just the right amount of the hormone thyroxine to keep things running smoothly. If the pipeline slows, your metabolism starts to crawl, says Eneida O.

Roldan, M.D., chair of the American Board of Bariatric Medicine.

It's normal for your thyroid to produce less thyroxine as you age, says Dr. Roldan. "That's why it's very important for women in their forties to do some kind of weight training," she says.

Progesterone. Produced in your ovaries during the second half of your menstrual cycle, progesterone actually boosts your body's ability to burn fat. It keeps your thyroid gland working properly and stabilizes blood sugar so that you're less likely to snack. But once progesterone levels take a nosedive, many other hormones, such as testosterone and thyroxine, are affected. Progesterone also helps your body burn fat. Less progesterone, less fat burning.

DHEA. Shortly after you reach age 20, this antiaging hormone also begins to diminish. By the time 40 rolls around, your body makes about half as much as it did. And that's a shame. The less DHEA you have, the slower your metabolism and the easier it is to put on weight, says Dr. Bruner.

What's more, DHEA stabilizes levels of insulin, the hormone that sweeps glucose out of your bloodstream and into your cells to be used as energy. Too little DHEA, too much insulin, which prevents your body from using fat stores and also increases your appetite.

Growth hormone. Like DHEA, growth hormone is abundant in your youth. It keeps your cells vigorous and active and maintains lean body mass, bone density, and a healthy muscle-to-fat ratio. But as you age and your supply plummets, so does your ability to burn calories without exercise. The muscle you lose gets replaced by fat, says Dr. Bruner.

With all these forces of nature working against you, it's tempting to just lie back and accept the inevitable. But just as you can control how much muscle you preserve—

and gain—through weight training, you can get your hormones back in sync with various therapies that only your physician can prescribe, including hormone replacement therapy and synthetic thyroid or growth hormones.

Responsibility Overload

In addition to our jobs, we're wives, mothers, chauffeurs, housekeepers, cooks, and accountants. Many of us also care for aging parents. That leaves very little time for ourselves. Going to an exercise class at the gym? Ha! About

Think Yourself Thin

"In our society, there are many negative messages about weight, willpower, and body image," says Lisa Talamini, R.D., director of program development and nutrition at Jenny Craig in La Jolla, California. To counter these external negatives and retrain your mindset, practice saying positive statements like these.

1. I can enjoy all my favorite foods in moderation.
2. I take the time to nourish my body.
3. Every time I eat a food, I enjoy its color, its taste, and its texture.
4. I can be more active today than I was yesterday.
5. Today I keep my body and my mind in balance.
6. I reward myself for every positive change I make in my life.
7. I live by choice, not by chance.
8. I am learning to love my body and myself.
9. I accept myself just as I am.
10. I ride the wave of my temptations.

as likely as taking a spur-of-the-moment vacation to the Bahamas.

Playing these different roles adds up to big-time stress, another contributor to weight gain. Chronic stress causes the body to release the hormone cortisol, which sends fat straight to the belly, says Dr. Roldan.

Even women who are full-time homemakers are at risk, says Dr. Roldan. They're more likely to experience depression and low self-esteem, which often lead to inactivity and overeating, she says. "Some homemakers may be totally dependent on their families for their self-worth, and that changes once the kids go off to college." The solution is to put yourself at the top of your list of things to do, and don't feel guilty about it. Care for yourself the way you care for your family. Set aside time to exercise and unwind when you know you won't be disturbed. If that means getting up before your family rises, so be it, says Dr. Roldan.

"Let's say your mom is in the hospital with a broken hip," says Dr. Peeke. "Go visit her. Get her the flowers. Spend time with her. Then get out to the gym for 20 to 30 minutes or walk briskly around the hospital grounds. You'll recharge your batteries, and you'll feel better."

The Dietary Checkup

With all the stress and time pressures in your life, grabbing an extra piece of chocolate, a bowl of ice cream, or a bag of potato chips soon becomes the norm. And if dinner isn't cooked, you're more likely to drive to the nearest fast-food restaurant. Eating out? That's a reward for all of your hard work. After all, you reason, "I deserve it."

But those calories add up, and so do the pounds. "Fast food is convenient but very high in fat. You neglect to eat your fruits and vegetables, and so does your family," says

Priscilla Clarkson, Ph.D., professor of exercise science at the University of Massachusetts in Amherst.

A food plan to help you cope with daily stress, strengthen your immune system, maintain muscle mass, and produce a gradual weight loss looks like this.

Nix refined carbohydrates. That includes white flour, white rice, white pasta, white potatoes, white bread, and table sugar, which is found in cookies, cakes, and sweetened cereals. Their high sugar content causes normal insulin levels to skyrocket, placing undue stress on your body. "Your insulin levels go up and down like a roller coaster," says Dr. Peeke. "And if this happens consistently, you risk developing diabetes down the line because your body is constantly dealing with a boatload of sugar and isn't releasing a steady flow of insulin—which you'd get by eating high-fiber foods."

Get the dark starches. Eat brown rice, whole wheat or spinach pasta, whole wheat bread, and sweet potatoes. Cook with monounsaturated fats, such as olive oil and canola oil, to strengthen your immune system. Choose low-fat protein, such as poultry, fish, and lean red meat. "Proteins are the building blocks of muscle, so these foods will preserve lean mass and bolster your metabolism," says Dr. Peeke.

Time your carbs. Eat your high-fiber starches before 5:00 P.M. Even though they're chock-full of nutrients, they're also high in calories, which means that they can prevent you from reaching your weight-loss goals. "You'll never lose weight faster than if you eliminate the starches after 5:00 P.M. Your weight will peel right off," says Dr. Peeke. That's because high-fiber starches like rice don't come in single-serving packages, so we're more likely to overeat.

Cut back on alcohol. While there isn't any fat in alcohol, it's loaded with calories that get stored as fat, says

Dr. Roldan. Gram for gram, alcohol provides more calories than carbohydrates or protein: One gram of fat supplies 9 calories; alcohol has 7, and carbohydrates and protein have 4 each. As if that weren't bad enough, drinking even moderate amounts can increase your appetite and cause you to lose control over how much you're eating. So stick with one alcohol serving a day, says Dr. Roldan. That's either a 12-ounce can of beer, 1½ ounces of hard liquor, or 5 ounces of wine. The best beverage for weight loss? Good old-fashioned water. It's fat- and calorie-free.

Finding Support

In 1998 and 1999, more than 750 residents of Dyersville, Iowa, joined together to lose weight. In 10 weeks, without using starvation or fad diets, they lost altogether a whopping 7,500 pounds.

Their secret: They gave one another lots of support.

From the groups of 6 to 10 that met weekly to the thumbs-up signs they got every day from everyone else in town (population 5,000), the weight-loss participants never felt that they had to walk the path to their goals alone.

While it's doubtful that we're going to get an entire town cheering us on every time we drop a pound, we can—and must—create our own support network to help us meet our goals.

"Your ability to get social support is every bit as critical as understanding the foods you eat and their fat content and getting yourself more physically active," says Susan J. Bartlett, Ph.D., assistant professor of medicine at Johns Hopkins Medical Institutions in Baltimore and a psychologist specializing in weight management.

You Can't Go It Alone

Research consistently shows that a buddy can help you keep to a low-fat diet, stick to an exercise program, and lose more weight than you would on your own. You're even more likely to eat your fruits and vegetables if you get support from coworkers.

A landmark study out of the University of California, Berkeley, compared 44 women who had regained lost weight with 30 women who had maintained their lower weight. Seventy percent of the maintainers had sought help from friends, family members, or professionals when they had had problems. Only 38 percent of the relapsers

Sabotage from the Ones You Love

Friends and family can undermine your weight-loss efforts in subtle ways like the following.

Snacking in front of you. Simply watching someone eat could trigger unplanned eating. Staying focused on your weight-loss goals may keep you from giving in. If you really can't take it, walk away. Consider asking others not to eat tempting foods in your presence.

Pushing food. Someone eats in front of you and insists that you have some as well. Think through what you're going to say ahead of time, such as, "No thanks. I'm trying to eat healthier."

Policing food. You reach for dessert only to encounter raised eyebrows. Such a judgmental attitude could encourage you to retaliate by eating even more. Remind others that you've made a lifestyle change, which is not the same thing as a strict diet.

Giving advice. They mean well, but their continual advice is annoying. Explain that everyone loses weight

had reached out. In fact, one-fourth of the relapsers had had no social support at all.

"Social support is one of the best predictors of how you're going to do with your weight loss in the long term," says Dr. Bartlett. The reason, she says, is that to make these kinds of lifestyle changes, you need a cheerleading squad.

"If you're a mother, for example, you need a family that's willing to support your making these changes, willing to give you time to exercise, and willing to make modifications in their food and their eating," Dr. Bartlett says.

her own way and that this program is what works for you.

Giving negative feedback. It's hard to stay confident when friends and family tell you that you can't lose weight. But people have power over you only if you give it to them.

Giving guilt. Others might be intimidated by your weight loss and could try to make you feel guilty. Assure them that you're the same person you've always been, and treat them the same way you always have.

Ignoring your progress. Remain positive by pointing out the small changes in your body and in the way you feel.

Encouraging you to skip exercise. Your exercise program may take time away from loved ones. If they feel left out, share activities with them, such as walks or bike rides.

Asking your weight. If you don't want to tell them, point out that good health is more important than numbers on a scale.

How Support Groups Help

Sharing your weight-loss goals with others in a group setting keeps you accountable and realistic, says Ruth Quillian, Ph.D., a psychologist at the Duke Center for Living in Durham, North Carolina. So it's more likely that you'll meet those goals. Because everyone is in the same situation, it is easier to find support and understanding in a safe and less critical environment. Here's how to make the most of group support.

Get help from experts. Try a program like Weight Watchers or TOPS. These groups have years of experience and thousands of success stories.

Lean on a leader. Negative thoughts and comments aren't necessarily banished once you walk into the room, but a leader can keep people's attitudes and comments positive.

Support can be particularly important in maintaining physical activity, says Susan Kayman, R.D., Dr.P.H., project manager of weight management programs for Kaiser Permanente's northern California region. "Some women have the internal drive to run on their own and go to the gym and work out on their own, but the majority of us are not like that. Women are very social beings, and one way to get more physical activity into your life is to make plans to exercise with someone else." Then focus on socialization, not just the activity. That means walking with a friend, driving to the gym with a friend, or meeting friends at the gym. Without that kind of support, she says, we're likely to just quit.

Bobbi Schell, who not only helped organize the Dyersville program but also participated in it, still meets a group of friends every Saturday morning at 6:30 to work

Meet weekly. The more often you surround yourself with support, the easier it will be to reach your goal.

Look for a lifestyle program. The program you join should set realistic goals and focus on overall lifestyle, not just pounds. If the program recommends that you eat fewer than 1,200 calories a day, find another one.

Exchange numbers. Find a few women to network with outside of meetings. Exchange e-mail addresses and phone numbers and keep in touch daily.

Stay active. Moving around is important, so look for a support group that encourages exercise and even organizes group activities.

Set goals for indulgence. Schedule massages, manicures, and bubble baths, and encourage the other women in your group to do the same.

out. "I schedule my life to make sure that I don't miss it; it's so nurturing," she says.

Would she do it on her own? "Never," says the rehab services outreach supervisor at Mercy Medical Center, St. Mary's Unit, the hospital that sponsored the weight-loss programs.

What Do You Need?

The type of support you need will determine the type of person you should get it from, says Kristine Kelsey, R.D., Ph.D., a research assistant professor of nutrition at the University of North Carolina in Chapel Hill. The four types:

Emotional support. You need someone to just be there and listen. This might be your best friend or partner.

Tangible support. You need someone to provide some assistance, like exercising with you, cooking with you, or going to the grocery store to help you shop differently. Look to friends, coworkers, or your partner.

Informational support. You need someone who shares articles and books she's read about weight loss or who provides simple education, like the number of calories in a piece of pie. This might be a nutritionist, doctor, or friend.

Appraisal support. You need someone who will tell you how great you're doing, encourage you, compliment you on your appearance. This may come from people you barely know in the office or neighborhood or from friends and relatives who know of your efforts.

You may need all four or just one. But whatever your needs, be sure to make them clear to the people you look to for support.

"That's the thing we're very, very poor at doing," says Dr. Bartlett. "We assume that everyone knows how to support us, but the truth is that what's helpful for me may not be helpful for you."

Ask yourself these questions: Do I need an exercise buddy? Someone to keep me away from the cookies and cake? Help avoiding the cake at office parties? Someone to watch the kids while I exercise? Someone to take over the grocery shopping so that I don't buy high-calorie snacks? Or someone to fix dinner so that I'm not constantly taste testing?

Then be clear and specific about your needs, says Dr. Bartlett. "You could say to your husband, 'One way you could be helpful to me is on Friday nights, when I'm too tired to cook, decide in advance what restaurant we're going to so we don't just hit the closest KFC,'" she says.

What doesn't work is depending on others who are supportive and helpful in the way *they* think you need, such as a friend who turns into the food police, constantly berating you: "Don't eat that; that's bad for you. That's too fattening."

"Don't choose them unless that's the kind of help you want," says Dr. Bartlett.

Choosing Your A-Team

What you're looking for are people who are going to cheerlead for you, help you through tough times, celebrate your successes, and understand your weaknesses.

"Do you have someone you can talk to when you have a problem? About things other than weight loss?" asks Dr. Kayman. "That may be the person you need."

Think twice before picking your husband as a support. Most of the maintainers in the University of California, Berkeley, study had to look outside the home, with more than half the women saying that their husbands were *not* supportive of their weight-loss efforts.

Some even sabotaged their wives' efforts.

The reasons this happens vary, says Barbara Jacobson, Ph.D., a Seattle-based psychologist and author of *Weight, Sex, and Marriage.*

Sometimes a husband is insecure and fears that if his wife loses weight, she'll have an affair or leave him. Or he's overweight himself and becomes anxious about how his wife will view him when she no longer is. Or he simply likes food, enjoys eating out, and fears the change that this weight-loss program will mean for *his* life.

There's another reason not to choose your spouse or partner for special support in weight loss: "Men just don't get it," says Dr. Jacobson. "Their weight is not a complex issue for them. They don't have their identity all tied up in it. So it's very hard for them to give the kind of sympathy and support that women may need."

There is an exception to the husband rule: If your husband is trying to lose weight, too, he could turn out to be a good ally. In one study comparing two groups—obese people who lost weight with their spouses and those who lost weight alone—the women who participated with their husbands did much better.

So where do you find social support? Basically, anywhere you can get it, says Dr. Bartlett. "It could even be a relative who lives 3,000 miles away who e-mails you. You just need someone who is reliable and who will be enthusiastic, encouraging, and positive for you."

That might even mean getting it from total strangers on the Internet. One study showed that dieters who received interactive guidance on the Internet—including weekly feedback via e-mail from a behavior modification expert and an online bulletin board to talk to others trying to reduce—lost more weight than those who got no support.

And don't forget coworkers.

"I see all kinds of examples of people at work being a support system for each other," says Dr. Bartlett. "It may start casually with one person mentioning that she wants to lose weight, and the other says that she does, too, and they start walking together at lunch 1 or 2 days a week. Eventually, they're walking 5 days a week and doing other things together, like bowling or eating dinner out."

One Town's Experience

In Dyersville, Iowa, the weight-loss participants held weekly team meetings. They set up e-mail lists to encourage one another, came up with team slogans, and set team goals, says Schell.

The team approach was critical to the program's success, Schell says. "There's safety in numbers. No one likes to think she's the only one that has a problem." For instance, people who never exercised before began working out in the Dyersville recreation center. "This way, they could go with nine other people on their team and look just like everyone else," she says.

In a postprogram survey, one woman said that she wouldn't eat a piece of chocolate because she didn't want to let her team down. "But if I were doing it alone, I'd go ahead and eat it."

This group approach is one reason weight-loss programs like TOPS and Weight Watchers are often so successful, says Dr. Bartlett.

The Wrong Reward: Chocolate

When Tammy Hansen, a science teacher in Rockford, Michigan, tried to lose weight, she discovered how difficult it was to get support from her husband.

She joined TOPS with a friend 7 years ago. They were both stay-at-home moms at the time and exercised or walked in the evenings. But when Tammy got home and faced her family, she found temptation everywhere, especially in her husband's "rewards" for losing weight: chocolate-covered raisins, her danger food.

"My husband is naturally thin and can eat whatever he wants without gaining weight," Tammy says. "He just doesn't understand how I struggle. So his idea of support is chocolate."

At first, Tammy accepted and ate his gifts, only to feel guilty about it later. She realized that she had to make her husband understand how much she needed his help. She told him over and over again that she couldn't lose weight on her own and that if there was chocolate in the house, she'd eat it.

It worked. With her husband's help, she lost 61 pounds and has kept it off for 7 years.

"When my patients come to see me, they get one view, one perspective, and one voice of encouragement. When they come to a group meeting, there are nine others sitting in that room going through the same thing that they're going through. Someone who has gone through a slump and come out the other end is going to have much more credibility than I have."

To supercharge a group's effectiveness, build it with friends. In one study, researchers compared the weight-loss success of two groups: those who joined a program with three friends and those who joined alone and were teamed with strangers. Ninety-five percent of the participants who joined with friends completed the 10-month program, compared with 76 percent of those who joined alone. Members of the "friends" teams also lost more weight.

Once you've identified potential supporters, keep in mind that a support system is not a one-way street. You have to give to get. That means saying "thank you," communicating honestly, and expressing your appreciation, maybe even with a small gift.

"The best social support system is one in which I support you on something, and in return you support me on something," says Dr. Bartlett. For instance, if your husband is supporting your weight-loss efforts and helps you find time for exercise, then you support his fly-fishing hobby and help him find time to go fishing or take a fly-making class.

The Kind of Support You Don't Need

There's positive support, and there's negative support—and sometimes it's hard to tell the difference. Like the husband who, when his wife lost 10 pounds, presented her with a box of chocolates.

It's called social sabotage. Dr. Kayman had one client whose neighbor would always bring over pies and other baked goods. "Because this woman didn't want to hurt her neighbor's feelings, she would eat the pie rather than clearly saying, 'This is the worst thing for me right now.'"

"We wouldn't think of offering a drink to a recovering alcoholic or giving a cigarette to someone who is trying to quit smoking, but we actually act offended when we offer people food and they turn us down because they're trying to lose weight," says Kristi Ferguson, Ph.D., associate professor of community and behavioral health at the University of Iowa College of Public Health in Iowa City.

That's when you need to be assertive and clearly express your feelings and needs, says Dr. Kayman. "Women often have great difficulty in being able to say what we need because we're so used to meeting the needs of others. Many relapsers are women who didn't feel like they deserved to be able to tell the other person what they needed; they didn't want to hurt the other person's feelings."

This isn't easy, and you may benefit from professional help to build up your assertiveness skills, she adds.

Remember, people can sabotage you only if you let them, says Karen Miller-Kovach, R.D., chief scientist at Weight Watchers International. "Sabotage is a two-way street. We all know food pushers, but I've never met one yet who literally shoves food down another person's throat. You have the right to say no and stick to it. A pleasant but firm statement that you will not comply with the saboteur's request almost always works."

Sometimes the negativity is more obvious. Dr. Bartlett hears constantly from women whose families and friends react to their weight-loss plans with a virtual roll of their eyes and the comment "Again? Why bother? How many times have you done this now?"

And sometimes the negative "support" comes in the form of jealousy, says Howard J. Rankin, Ph.D., behavioral psychology advisor for the TOPS Club and author of *7 Steps to Wellness*. People say, "You're getting too thin," when you've lost only a couple of pounds.

Deal with these naysayers by understanding that each of us views life through our own lens, says Dr. Rankin. "You shouldn't be deflected from your goal because of other people's neuroses."

Maintaining
the New You

You're so good. You've spurned short-term "diets" in favor of healthy living, learned to practice portion control, and incorporated exercise and other physical activity into your daily life. Now you even recognize your emotional eating triggers. You've lost 20 pounds, and you feel and look terrific. By all rights, you should be resting on your laurels.

Well, don't even think about relaxing. The toughest part is still ahead.

With 75 percent of dieters who are not physically active regaining, within 1 to 2 years, the weight that they lost, maintaining your weight loss may prove one of your greatest challenges. But that doesn't mean that it can't be done.

From examining hundreds of women who have been successful not only at losing weight but at keeping it off, some weight-loss experts have identified two key traits: permanent behavior change centered on health, not appearance, and old self-image changed to accurately reflect the new, slimmer reality.

Diets Fade, Health Is Forever

"If a woman has gone on a diet to get a boyfriend or to wear a size 6, she's likely to go back to her old habits once she loses the weight," says Fugen Neziroglu, Ph.D., senior clinical director of the Bio-Behavioral Institute in Great Neck, New York. If, however, her goal was to improve her overall health, with losing weight an almost unintended consequence, she's more likely to keep that weight off.

"One of the critical findings," says Anne Fletcher, R.D., of the 160 weight-loss maintainers she interviewed for her book *Thin for Life*, "was that they stopped seeing what they did to lose the weight as separate from what they

Don't Weigh Yourself Every Day

Your weight fluctuates daily, and the number on the scale may have nothing to do with how much you actually weigh or with how much fat you've lost or gained. The variables are the time of day, the clothes you wear, and what you ate or drank the night before. Fluid retention can also make your weight seesaw by as much as 4 pounds in a single day.

Weekly changes in weight are more significant, but you can still have variations that don't reflect a true picture. You may have a significant loss one week and then have a ½-pound gain the next, but monthly weighing should show an overall loss if you're sticking to a healthy weight-loss program.

Your menstrual cycle has an impact on fluid retention and weight. You may lose weight for a few weeks,

needed to do to keep it off. And in losing the weight for good, they took the focus off 'dieting' and put it on permanently adopting a healthy lifestyle."

There are many lessons that we can learn from their success.

Plan for problems. Even when a patient is doing well maintaining her weight, Cathy Nonas, R.D., director of the VanItallie Center for Nutrition and Weight Management in New York City, still works with her to anticipate problems.

Maybe the woman roams the kitchen after dinner. Today she's snagging "good" snacks like rice cakes or carrots, but tomorrow it might be pie or ice cream. Some questions that Nonas explores include: Why is she in the kitchen at all? And why does she feel compelled to eat after dinner? Once the woman can answer those ques-

then see either a smaller loss, a plateau, or even a slight gain the week before or during menstruation. This is normal. The loss will continue when your period ends.

While you shouldn't weigh yourself every day, neither should you ignore the scale. Often, women go into psychological denial about their weight, choosing not to recognize that they have been overeating and are gaining weight. What works best for most women is to weigh themselves weekly but to focus on monthly progress.

Expert consulted: Laurie L. Friedman, Ph.D., deputy director, Johns Hopkins Weight Management Center, Baltimore

tions, Nonas works with her to develop alternatives so that she can avoid this weak spot. Some alternatives would be to not go into the kitchen after dinner, change her usual habits by exercising in the evening, or eat dinner slightly later.

You can do the same thing. List potential weak spots when you're likely to fall into your old habits, like snacking when you watch TV or tasting when you're cooking, and then think of a solution to your problem. Solutions may include staying out of the kitchen while you watch TV or chewing gum while you're cooking to cut down on tasting.

Say okay to imperfection. One common element of weight maintenance that Fletcher found in her 160 weight-loss "masters" was that they gave themselves permission to not be perfect. Who wants to go through life never again eating ice cream or chocolate or potato chips? "It's fine to eat those foods from time to time and in moderation," she says.

So when you crave a chocolate bar, buy one, eat a little, and freeze the rest. We often desire just the taste of something, says Jeannette F. Jordan, R.D., prevention/detection education coordinator at the Medical University of South Carolina in Charleston. If you try to fulfill the craving with something like a sandwich or crackers, you'll still yearn for chocolate, she says. And if you eat the chocolate anyway, you'll have consumed more calories than you might have with just the candy.

Get real: your real weight. Often, overweight people set fantasy goal weights that are very difficult to maintain, says Fletcher. About one-third of her weight-loss subjects accepted themselves at a somewhat heavier weight than their original goal. "One woman, who is 5 feet 8 inches tall, got down to 140 pounds and felt like she was living in a cage, obsessing about every mouthful and exercising fanatically," she says. When the woman took a reality break and accepted a healthy (for her) weight in the 150s, she was much happier.

Be a journalist. Food journals can be an important tool to achieve weight loss. They keep you aware of what you're eating and may reveal hidden calories that you didn't even realize are in your diet, says Suzanne W. Dixon, R.D., a research epidemiologist and registered dietitian at the Henry Ford Health System in Detroit. If you tracked your foods while you were dropping the pounds, don't drop your pen and notebook when you've achieved your goal weight. "You need to periodically see where your calories are coming from to nip any problems in the bud," says Dixon.

Stay in touch with the scale. Most of Fletcher's weight losers reported that regular self-weighing—at least once a week—was an important element of long-term success. "It keeps you accountable," she says.

Report in monthly. Each month, ask yourself: Have I been eating enough vegetables? Is my eating style something I can do for the rest of my life and not feel like it's a punishment? Is my activity level as high as it should be? Am I healthier?

Keep moving. In a study of weight maintainers versus regainers, researchers found that those who maintained their loss reported lots of physical activity; more than half said that they worked up a sweat at least three times per week. Just 30 percent of regainers reported that level of activity.

Reward yourself. Treat yourself for maintaining your weight. Whether it's catching a movie or buying a new CD, these personal incentives will remind you that you're doing great.

Match Mental Images

One key to lasting weight control is in the mind. If understanding the connection between eating and our emotions was important when we were losing the weight, it's doubly so now.

Dance the Night Away

Can the samba keep you slim? Yes. A night on the dance floor gives you a workout and enhances your social life.

"If you're dancing socially all evening, you're getting a sustained low-impact aerobic workout," says Jackie Rogers, director of dance and exercise for the National Dance Council of America (NDCA). An hour of ballroom dancing is the equivalent of a low-impact aerobics class.

The most rigorous dances? Polka, swing, and quickstep. In swing particularly, which has enjoyed a resurgence, you get "wonderful exercise," Rogers says. "You're moving more because you're kicking your legs and making motions that you don't do in the fox-trot or waltz."

Socially, dancing is a great way to foster togetherness—or to find some. A night on the dance floor is a romantic activity for couples, Rogers says. And dance studios often have group classes that students attend solo, finding partners from the class.

To start dancing, check out classes at local adult education programs, colleges, and commercial dance studios. Look for certified instructors who have qualifications from a member organization of the National Dance Council of America, the governing body for dance professionals in the United States. For additional information, you can contact the NDCA at (800) 291-8623.

But the mental connection doesn't stop there. Now that we've changed our bodies through weight loss, it's important to let our minds catch up to our new selves. "Many women come to me after losing 30 to 40 pounds and putting it right back on, over and over," says Sally Ann Greer, Ph.D., a psychologist in Arlington, Virginia. The problem is that their self-images are stuck in the "fat" position. "When they lose the weight, there's a conflict between that inner image and the actual image in the mirror."

In an effort to make the two images match, we change our behaviors back again, says Dr. Greer. "We'll take the second helpings and not pay attention to portion size. We decrease our exercise and gradually put the weight back on."

The remedy is a "tincture of time," says Jan McBarron, M.D., director of Georgia Bariatrics, a medical center for overweight people in Columbus, Georgia, and cohost of the nationally syndicated health talk show *Duke and the Doctor*. "If you don't take a full 18 months to change your self-image, your weight comes right back."

Photographs are a great way to flip the switch, says Dr. Neziroglu. At her clinic, she asks patients to compare before-and-after snapshots. Then Dr. Neziroglu asks the women about the traits or qualities ascribed to the different pictures. "When women look at the 'before' pictures, they may have such negative images that they call themselves disgusting," she says. Even when they see the "after" photos, some women still don't view themselves as being thinner. "They might say, 'I still look fat' or 'I look better,' but rarely does someone declare, 'You know, I look good.'"

Here's how to help your inner image of yourself match your outer image.

Talk to yourself. While looking at your reflection in a mirror or while gazing at a photo of your slimmed-down self, utter positive statements like "I like myself at this weight," "I am a good person regardless of my weight, but I prefer this weight for health reasons," "I feel confident that I am in control of my weight," and "I don't need to eat to cope with life."

Go easy on yourself. Because self-criticism and moral judgments about eating are so prevalent with overweight women, Dr. McBarron advises kindness—to yourself. "Do I still eat desserts occasionally, drink wine sometimes, and overeat? Sure I do," says the physician, who lost 70 pounds herself. "Do I beat myself up and feel guilty? No." Keeping weight off, she says, is a process, not a destination.

Update your inner image. Through the power of self-hypnosis—it induces a profoundly relaxed yet aware state—Dr. Greer urges patients to mentally see themselves at their new weight just as others physically see them. "Try to involve as many senses as you can in this imagery: How does it feel physically to be at this weight? How does it look? How does it feel emotionally?" The idea is to replace that erroneous but stubborn inner image with an accurate one. An audiotape such as *Edgar Cayce: Self-Hypnosis* will teach you the proper technique.

Dr. Greer also recommends consulting with a psychologist who is trained in self-hypnosis. To find someone in your area, send a self-addressed, stamped envelope to the American Society of Clinical Hypnosis, 33 West Grand Avenue, Suite 402, Chicago, Illinois 60610, and request a list of the psychologists in your local area who are trained in teaching self-hypnosis to help maintain weight loss.

Dress to thrill. Many women who have been overweight won't allow themselves a lot of jewelry, makeup, or dressy clothes, even when they trim down, says Dr. Neziroglu, because they still have their old belief that these trappings won't make any difference. So she assigns her clients homework: Go shopping. She encourages them to buy clothes in their new sizes and accessorize with jewelry, scarves, and shoes. "It changes the way they see

She Avoids the "Three Cs" to Maintain Weight Loss

When Roe Wiersgalla joined TOPS, in 1997, she weighed 336 pounds. Now 146 pounds lighter, this Milwaukee office manager found a foolproof way to triumph over temptation.

"My downfall was the Three Cs: cookies, candy, and cake. I absolutely love them. I managed to control my urge for them the first time I dropped a lot of weight, after TOPS. When I got to my recommended weight, my doctor said I shouldn't lose any more. I began to gradually eat more and more of the Three Cs.

"It was as though I had permission to indulge— until the day I ate 5,000 calories in sugar. I panicked. I knew if I kept up at that rate, in just a few months I could put all that weight back on. So I resolved to make certain things completely taboo and not have even a taste.

"Now I treat sugar like an alcoholic treats liquor. The big hurdle is the first decision: 'Am I having the sugar or not?'—and I'm not. I won't even lick my fingers when I serve pastry to others. When I see plates of cookies at a party now, my response is automatic: I give them no consideration whatsoever. I feel absolutely in control of my irresistible temptation.

"I may have more of some other foods from time to time, but when it comes to those Three Cs, I just have zero. That really works for me."

themselves," she says. "For the first time in a long time, they feel attractive—and know they can feel this way regardless of their weight."

Techniques for Tough Times

A fight with your husband. A job promotion. Your teenager's failing grades. Next thing you know, you're standing in front of the refrigerator, slathering mayonnaise on thick slices of bologna and stuffing them into your mouth.

The stress of both positive and negative change can trigger relapses, says Susan M. Ice, M.D., medical director of the Renfrew Center of Philadelphia, which specializes in eating disorders and women's mental health issues. Women, Dr. Ice says, are particularly vulnerable to emotional stress.

Here's how to manage through these tough times without reverting to old, unhealthy habits.

Quiz yourself. Ask these basic questions: Am I hungry? Thirsty? Tired? Do I need a cookie—or a walk? Am I present for my meal, or am I allowing my emotions to distract me? Questions as simple as these can help you refocus on yourself, says Lisa Talamini, R.D., director of program development and nutrition at Jenny Craig in La Jolla, California.

Take time for you. Just as you block time on your calendar for appointments, schedule time for physical activity, grocery shopping, writing in your journal, or even just taking a bubble bath.

Surround yourself with support. Return to your weight-maintenance support group, advisor, or buddy to share your fears, struggles, and issues. This is also the time to make sure that those close to you know that you need support, says Roxanne E. Moore, R.D., nutrition education coordinator at Towson University in Baltimore and spokeswoman for the American Dietetic Association. That way, your husband will know that you won't snap at him if he comments on your hand in the cookie jar. And his supportive words—"Honey, you seem to be going for cookies lately. What's really on your mind?"—could be just the release you need to close that jar.

Step back. If you find yourself slipping, say to yourself, "Okay, I'm engaging in old habits because . . . ," and fill in the blank, says Dr. Neziroglu. "The answer might be 'because my boss gave me a hard time, I'm feeling worthless, and I must have everyone's approval all the time.'" Challenging that erroneous thought—that you must be thought well of by everyone, always—will help you see the troubling situation realistically so you can resume healthy eating.

Write it down. A personal journal that emphasizes feelings—not activities—helps women keep in touch with themselves, says Dr. Ice. That self-checking is critical to staying balanced when you're tempted to tip back into old habits. The personal journal can be part of the food journal discussed earlier in this chapter.

Relapse Remedies

Oops! That muffled thud is the sound of you falling off the healthy-eating wagon. It happens to the best of us, but it doesn't mean that you can't pick yourself up, brush off the dust, and climb back aboard.

"One of the key predictors of success in weight maintenance is how you handle a slip," says Howard J. Rankin, Ph.D., behavioral psychology advisor for the TOPS Club and author of *7 Steps to Wellness*. "You can use it as an excuse to say that you can't stay on track, so why bother. Or you can recognize that it happens to everyone, and you can rebound positively from it."

Try to react positively, not punitively, if you've had a lapse, says Talamini. "The old, negative cycle would be to feel guilty, mentally beat yourself up, and drastically restrict your eating. What works, though, is tuning up your skills to take better care of yourself."

Here's how.

Work the numbers. If you fall off the maintenance bandwagon for one day or a couple, before you start berating yourself, look at the calendar, says Dr. McBarron. "There are 30 days in a month. If you have stuck with your healthy living habits for 25 days, you're way ahead of the game."

Develop fast reflexes. If pounds start reappearing, don't wait to respond. It's easier to lose 5 pounds than 10.

Set self-boundaries. Determine in advance your "manageable range" of weight fluctuation, and have a plan to handle it. For example, if you've gained 5 pounds, you'll boost your broth intake to fill up before meals or change the ratio of low-calorie foods to higher-calorie foods by adding more steamed vegetables and reducing the amount of meat. At 10 extra pounds, you'll go back to support group meetings or check in with your doctor or nutritionist, says Nonas.

Remember why you did this. "People often need to face a fearful situation before committing to making lifestyle changes. For example, seeing one of her parents die from a heart attack or being told that she has diabetes and may suffer other health problems if she doesn't lose weight is often all a woman needs to hear to start making positive behavior changes," says Moore. Write down your reasons and post them on the refrigerator door as a daily in-your-face reminder of why you wanted to feel good.

Plan for problems. Since haphazard eating is a major cause of weight gain, go on relapse-alert status when your routine changes. An imminent holiday or trip is a signal to think about how you'll handle upcoming meals and temptations. To prevent any problems, Dr. Ice makes these suggestions.

- Structure mealtimes by eating at the same time every day.
- Have a plan that includes other "nourishing" things to do at high-risk times, like taking a walk, reading, writing in your journal, talking to a friend, or playing a game.
- Don't eat meals alone.

Index